The Christian Virtues in Medical Practice

The Christian Virtues in Medical Practice

Edmund D. Pellegrino
David C. Thomasma

WITH THE EDITORIAL ASSISTANCE OF
David G. Miller

Georgetown University Press / Washington, D.C.

Georgetown University Press, Washington, D.C.

Printed in the United States of America

10 9 8 7 6 5 4 3 2 1996

THIS VOLUME IS PRINTED ON ACID-FREE OFFSET BOOK PAPER

Library of Congress Cataloging-in-Publication Data

Pellegrino, Edmund D.,
The Christian virtues in medical practice / Edmund D. Pellegrino, David C. Thomasma
P. cm.
Includes bibliographical references.
1. Medical ethics. 2. Christian ethics. 3. Cardinal virtues.
I. Thomasma, David C. II. Title
R725.56.P45 1996
174'.2—dc20
ISBN 0-87840-566-6 94-11007

To our teachers, those Dominicans, Jesuits, and Vincentians who tried to instill in us the congruence of faith and reason that has characterized the Catholic intellectual tradition for centuries. For fidelity to that tradition, we thank them; for any lapse, we remain responsible. We also thank our many role models whose qualities prompted us to write this book. Many have shared their faith and taught us through their lives and demeanor the infinite variety of goodness and mercy.

For it seems to me that the first responsibility of the man of faith is to make his faith really part of his own life, not by rationalizing it, but living it.

—Thomas Merton, *No Man Is an Island* (New York: Harcourt, Brace, 1955), p. xiv.

Contents

Acknowledgments

We wish to thank Marti Patchell and Doris Thomasma for their help in making the arrangements that brought about this book, as well as Travis Schwab for help in finding references and checking the text. We also thank the staff of the National Reference Center for Bioethics Literature, particularly Patricia Milmoe McCarrick; John Samples, Director of Georgetown University Press; and the staff of Loyola University Chicago, for their hospitality and graciousness. We are also grateful to the donors of the Fr. Michael I. English, S.J., Chair for their support, which enabled us to do the research and writing for this book. Special thanks goes to the Rev. J.D. Cassidy, O.P., who made many helpful suggestions for clarifying our ideas. We wish to thank him for the generosity of his time and his careful cogitation of our premises and conclusions.

Portions of some chapters previously appeared as articles. They have been substantially revised for this book:

Chapter One: Edmund D. Pellegrino, "Thomas Percival, the Ethics beneath the Etiquette," forward to *Medical Ethics; or, A Code of Institutions and Precepts Adapted to the Professional Conduct of Physicians and Surgeons,* by Thomas Percival [Reprinted from the 1805 version] (Birmingham, Ala.: Classics of Medicine Library, 1985), pp. 1–65. And Edmund D. Pellegrino, "Percival's Medical Ethics: The Moral Philosophy of an 18th-Century English Gentleman," *Archives of Internal Medicine* 146 (November 1986): 2265–2269; reprinted in *The Persisting Osler II: Selected Transactions of the American Osler Society 1981–1990,* ed. J.A. Barondess and C.G. Roland (Malabar, Fla.: Krieger, 1994), pp. 9–21.

Chapter Two: Edmund D. Pellegrino, "Health Care: A Vocation to Justice and Love," in *The Professions in Ethical Context: Vocations to Justice,* ed. Francis A. Eigo [Proceedings—Theology Institute of Villanova University] (Villanova, Pa.: Villanova University Press, 1986), pp. 97–126.

Chapter Three: Edmund D. Pellegrino and David C. Thomasma, "Autonomy and Trust in the Clinical Encounter: Reflections from a Theological Perspective," in *Theology and Medicine: Theology Analyses of the Clinical Encounter* [Vol. 3], ed. Gerald P. McKenny and Jonathan R. Sande (Dordrecht, Netherlands: Kluwer, 1994), pp. 69–84. And David C. Thomasma, "The Basis of Medicine and Religion: Respect for Persons," *Linacre Quarterly* 45, no. 2 (1980): 142–150.

Chapter Four: Edmund D. Pellegrino, "The Trials of Job: A Physician's Meditation," *Linacre Quarterly* 56, no. 2 (1989): 76–88.

Chapter Five: Edmund D. Pellegrino, "The Fact of Illness and the Act of Profession: Some Notes on the Source of Professional Obligation" (presentation at the Centennial Academic Assembly at Texas A&M University, Sept 16–17, 1976), in *Implications of History and Ethics to Medicine–Veterinary and Human,* ed. Laurence B. McCullough and James Polk Morris, III (College Station, Tex.: Texas A&M University, 1978), pp. 78–89. Edmund D. Pellegrino, "Health Care: A Vocation to Justice and Love," in *The Professions in Ethical Context: Vocations to Justice,* ed. Francis A. Eigo [Proceedings—Theology Institute of Villanova University] (Villanova, Pa.: Villanova University Press, 1986), pp. 97–126. And Edmund D. Pellegrino, "Beyond Bioethics: The Christian Obligation of Christian Physicians," in *Linking The Human Life Decisions,* ed. Russell Hittinger (Chicago: Regnery Gateway, 1986), pp. 143–167.

INTRODUCTION

Being a Christian Physician: Does It Make a Difference?

There are two very disturbing questions abroad today in the medical profession. One asks, "What difference does it make to be a physician?" The second asks, "What difference does it make to be a Christian physician?"

Corollaries of the first question are: Why should physicians be expected to adhere to a system of ethics that requires more of them than of other persons in our society? Why should physicians try to suppress self-interest, at great cost to their own welfare and that of their families, when other professionals pursue self-interest with singular determination? We addressed these questions philosophically in earlier works.[1] There we argued that the nature of the healing relationship is in itself the foundation for the special obligations of physicians as physicians. These obligations, we hold, are binding on all physicians.

In this book we turn our attention to the second question: what difference does it make to be a Christian physician? This question asks whether anything is required over and above what is derivable philosophically if one professes to be a Christian as well as a physician. This is a timely question, since many Christian physicians are unclear about their identity and behavior and about how to reconcile profession and faith in a secular, pluralistic society.

Christian physicians today too often separate their religious from their professional commitments. Some fear that too overt a commitment to Christian ethics would lead to imposition of the doctor's beliefs on the patient. Physicians have to be particularly sensitive to this danger, as any serious illness and its healing so often involve a spiritual crisis.[2] Seriously ill persons are exquisitely vulnerable, and exploitable physically and emotionally. It is distressing even to think that a physician would exploit a patient's illness to proselytize. One hopes that physicians would appreciate that the best way to evidence one's Christianity is by genuine commitment to the sick and the poor.

On the other hand, to distance oneself from one's fundamental beliefs and values is morally dangerous. Especially is this so in a pluralistic society, where public policy follows on public opinion shaped less by civil debate than by media pundits more committed to delivering the spectacular than to engaging in cogent inquiry. To be silent about one's beliefs is to impoverish this debate and to lose it by default. To suppress the religious perspective means tacitly to accept secular and civic religion as the final determinants of morality. To be sure, there is no such thing as a Christian, Jewish, or Islamic medicine. But this does not mean that being a Christian, Jew, or Moslem is irrelevant to being a physician. The Christian infuses healing with the spirit of the Word, the Jew with the Torah, and the Moslem with the Koran. The Christian physician is not just a physician who happens to be a Christian. He is, at once, a Christian and a physician, one who is competent, but one whose competence is practiced within the constraints of Christian ethics.

Christian physicians fail in their obligations if they do not give witness in private and public life to the way the values of the Gospel can and do transform their lives. Not to fuse belief and practice is to deny the special transformation of human life the Gospels announce. Then the issue is how, in a pluralistic society, the Christian physician can remain both Christian and a physician, acting charitably toward those who do not share his or her view but simultaneously responding to Christ's invitation: "Come, follow me."

Our aim in this book is to build upon the ethical obligations we derived on philosophical grounds in a companion volume on the virtues in medicine,[3] and to examine how those virtues are transformed when healing is raised to the level of Christian commitment and grace. Our emphasis will be on the kind of person a Christian physician ought to be. Thus, we will take the perspective of a virtue-based ethics, employing the conjunction of natural and supernatural ethics so eloquently and perceptively outlined in the *Secunda Secundae* of Thomas Aquinas' *Summa Theologiae*. There St. Thomas extended the Aristotelian theory of the natural virtues, intellectual and moral, into the supernatural realm open to Christian believers through revelation. In essence, this part of St. Thomas' teaching provides a sketch of what kind of person a Christian ought to be.

There is a new openness to the ethics of virtue today. This openness stems in part from the successes as well as the deficiencies of principles. These deficiencies have been exposed by the emergence of rival theories based in caring, virtue, experience of illness, casuistry, feminism, and moral psychology. They are exposed, too, by the experiences of ethicists in the clinical setting, where it is obvious that the way principles are interpreted, ordered, and applied depends on the character of the participants—physicians, patients, nurses, families, etc. The end result is not that we must abandon principles but that we must refine them and relate them to other sources of moral norms. This book, like our previous book, focuses on the kind of persons we ought to be as well as the kind of decisions we ought to make.

Efforts to combine a virtue ethic with principled ethical theories are laudable but have so far been less than successful. Beauchamp and Childress have made a serious attempt, but in the end they largely concentrate on the principles.[4] They do point out that a virtue theory has a special place in moral deliberation on health care, but argue that it cannot replace duty-based ethics: "The special role of virtues in ethical theory should not be construed as evidence for a primary role, as if a virtue-based theory were more important than or could replace obligation-based theories. The two kinds of theory have different emphases, but they are compatible and mutually reinforcing."[5] James Drane and William Ellos make a stronger case than this for the place of virtues in medical ethics.[6] A brief sketch of virtue theory in our first chapter will help develop this point.

Our approach differs in one important respect from those we have mentioned. Other efforts link virtue theory with principle-based theories without moving through the virtue of prudence—i.e., establishing right reason in action, *recta ratio agibilium,* as St. Thomas called it.[7] Moreover, other theories neglect the intrinsic relationship between prudence, the other virtues, and the nature of medicine and professional dedication. Thus, virtue- and principle-based theories in medical ethics must be closely linked with the nature of medicine itself—i.e., with a philosophy of medicine. This we have explored in other volumes. This volume concentrates on what might be, in fuller development, a theology of medical ethics.

In addition, a contemporary comprehensive theory of medical ethics would have to incorporate into the ethics of care, narrative ethics, and moral psychology valuable insights from the rebirth of casuistry. We do not attempt anything so ambitious in this book. To do so would be a task beyond our capabilities but one that appears to be an increasing necessity.

This volume proceeds through the theological virtues of faith, hope, and charity to the practical virtues such as prudence, justice, and compassion. Charity, love of one's neighbor, is the ordering virtue of Christian ethics, medical and otherwise. It should shape the whole of the healing relationship. Faith, hope, and compassion (like trust, which we discuss in our other volume on the philosophical analysis of virtues in medicine) are virtues intrinsic to the healing relationship, as are compassion, integrity, and respect for the patient as well as other health professionals.

A Christian commitment, if it is faithfully and fully present in a health professional, transforms that profession into a vocation. It raises the profession to a level of grace. Finally, if we are to remain faithful to being both Christian and professional, we must confront the growing problem of how to live with these commitments in a secular and pluralistic society. These problems occupy the concluding chapters.

Edmund D. Pellegrino, M.D.
Washington, D.C.

David C. Thomasma, Ph.D.
Chicago, Ill.

NOTES

1. Edmund D. Pellegrino and David C. Thomasma, *A Philosophical Basis of Medical Practice* (New York: Oxford University Press, 1981); *For the Patient's Good: The Restoration of Beneficence in Health Care* (New York: Oxford University Press, 1988).

2. Edmund D. Pellegrino and David C. Thomasma, *Medicine per vocazione: Impegno religioso in medicina*, trans. Antonio Puca (Rome: Editiones Dehoniane, 1994); forthcoming English version: *Helping and Healing* (Washington: Georgetown University Press, 1996).

3. Edmund D. Pellegrino and David C. Thomasma, *The Virtues in Medical Practice* (New York: Oxford University Press, 1993).

4. Tom L. Beauchamp and James F. Childress, *Principles of Biomedical Ethics*, 4th ed. (New York: Oxford University Press, 1994), pp. 462–508.

5. Beauchamp and Childress, *Principles of Biomedical Ethics*, p. 379.

6. James Drane, *Becoming a Good Doctor: The Place of Virtue and Character in Medical Ethics* (Kansas City, Mo.: Sheed & Ward, 1988); and William Ellos, *Ethical Practice in Clinical Medicine* (New York: Routledge, 1990).

7. For St. Thomas, an act is moral if it is capable of being controlled by an agent's will. The possibility of freedom being ordered by truth must exist for an act to be moral; that is, ordering of reason is required to direct an act to good moral ends (St. Thomas Aquinas, *Summa Theologiae* [Vol. 16], trans. and

ed. Thomas Gilby [New York: Blackfriars, 1969], I-II, q. 1–5, pp. 1–155). For Aquinas, the end determines the species of the moral act. This means that the end (sometimes the intention, sometimes the physical end of the action, sometimes the goal of the agent, sometimes all of the above) establishes the nature of the moral act itself, not necessarily the rectitude of the action, which is also subject to analysis in terms of other factors (objective evil of the act, extenuating circumstances, and the like). See Brian Mullady, *The Meaning of the Term "Moral" in St. Thomas Aquinas* (Vatican City: Libreria Editrice Vaticana, 1986).

1

Virtue-Based Ethics: Natural and Theological

Indeed, it is not learning that makes a man holy and just, but a virtuous life makes him pleasing to God.

—Thomas à Kempis, *The Imitation of Christ*, chapter 1

THE NATURAL VIRTUES

In a previous and companion work, we examined the place of the natural virtues in the moral life of medicine and the other health professions.[1] The natural virtues are those ascertainable by the use of human reason alone, unaided by scriptural revelation. They are defined in the new *Catechism* as "stable dispositions of the intellect and the will that govern our acts, order our passions, and guide our conduct."[2] In this volume our attention focuses on the supernatural virtues, those that are known through the Scriptures of the Jewish and Christian Bibles and the teachings of fathers and doctors of the Catholic Church.[3] The latter are the natural virtues now governing conduct through reason and faith combined. The *Catechism* defines them thus: "The theological virtues dispose Christians to live in a relationship with the Holy Trinity. They have God for their origin, their motive, and their object—God known by faith, God hoped in and loved for his own sake."[4]

Both the natural and the supernatural virtues are parts of what have now come to be called virtue ethics. As a propaedeutic to our discussion of the supernatural virtues, this chapter examines the history of virtue in moral thought and the current debates about where virtue ethics fits in contemporary ethical theory.

The classical quest of ethics was to find, and teach, the good life and how to live it. This was the common task of philosophers as diverse as Plato, Aristotle, Augustine, Aquinas, the Stoics, Confucius, the Hindu sages, and Lao-tsu. Different though their reasoning might be, they shared the convictions that it is in the nature of human beings to seek the good and that happiness and a good moral life are somehow synonymous. To be a good person and to live a good life were seen as aspirations of being human. These aspirations are not imposed on human beings but arise from their very nature as individuals and as social beings.

The classical quest for the good person and the good society presupposed a metaphysics of the good and a philosophical anthropology, as well as an objective order of morality ascertainable by human reason. It also presupposed role models in society. Ethics defined the kind of person one ought to be, and that was the virtuous person, the one habitually inclined to do the right and the good thing, no matter what the circumstances might be. Moral principles and moral reasoning were not neglected, but they were always grounded in some notion of the good as an end for human life; that end might be human happiness and fulfillment, as it was for Aristotle, or salvation, the redeemed community, and union with God, as it was for Thomas Aquinas.

The definition of virtue, the virtues, and the virtuous person has occupied philosophers since Plato first raised the question of virtue, its nature, number, and teachability.[5] Despite numerous efforts since then, no one has improved on Aristotle's imperfect but still useful definition. Aristotle identifies moral virtues as states of character, by which he means "the things in virtue of which we stand well or badly with reference to the passions."[6] Virtue is a particular state of character, one that "both brings into good condition the thing of which it is the excellence and makes the work of that thing be done well."[7] And further, "the virtue of a man also will be the state of character which makes a man good and which makes him do his work well."[8]

Implicit in Aristotle's definitions are several crucial ideas. First, virtues are, as they were for Socrates, excellences (*aretai*). They have a functional and teleological character, since they make things do their work well (cutting, in the case of a knife, and seeing, in the case of an eye, are Aristotle's examples) and by that fact make the thing itself good. They are intellectual when their end is truth and moral when their end is the good life. The good person learns them by practice and is guided in their use by practical wisdom.

Within these basic structures, Aristotle recognized the importance of ethical quandaries, conflicts of obligations, and the duties specific to certain stations in life. But quandaries were resolved in different terms than they are today. They were resolved in terms of the virtues one must possess—i.e., proper dispositions to the good. Thus, problems were not the center of ethical concern. Rather, they were the arena wherein the virtuous person exhibited the good way to live and to die. By learning how virtuous persons confronted moral dilemmas and by modeling after them, others could learn how to lead a good life. The communitarian origin and end of virtue theory is essential, since individuals are to be shaped by the virtues of the community within which they live. In their turn, those virtues need a community of belief if they are to be preserved and taught. In the Politics, Aristotle defined the good society that would sustain the virtues and also permit the virtuous person to flourish. St. Augustine and St. Thomas Aquinas, as we shall show later, expanded and completed the Aristotelian theory of virtue by adding to it the idea of the theological, or supernatural, virtues. These will be the major focus of the rest of this book.

The Aristotelian-Thomist concept of virtue began to change when philosophers of the Enlightenment challenged the metaphysical presuppositions of classical and medieval virtue ethics. The ideas of human nature, of a definable good as the end of human existence, and of an authority structure whence morality itself drew its binding force were called into question or denied outright. Faith was placed in human reason, not in divine law, as the source of morality. The center of gravity of ethics shifted from the kind of person one ought to be to the kind of decisions one ought to make, from the virtues one should cultivate to the principles, duties, and rules one ought to respect. Rules or principles were compelling in themselves or compelling because they guaranteed a good outcome, defined in terms of utility, harms, or goods.

In every age, societal issues must be evaluated from some framework. But now the shift had occurred from the individual, shaped by the community, to the instilling of virtues grounded in the power to persuade the reason. Perhaps this was an inevitable consequence of the post-Enlightenment breakdown of the power of the community and the church. As these community bonds dissolved, an appeal had to be made to principles that were supposed to transcend the beliefs of particular communities.

Ethical discourse moved with Kant, Mill, Hume, and Bentham from a primary focus on how the good person should act to a primary focus on how to resolve moral conflicts posed in difficult moral choices. Remnants of the classical medieval idea of an identifiable human nature remained with Hume, Hutcheson, Adam Smith, and Kant. But their definitions of virtue varied with the presuppositions of their philosophical systems. The questions these philosophers raised about the classical tradition shifted the focus ultimately from virtue to principles and duties. Rather than defining normative principles and duties by reference to the actions and character of the virtuous person, the virtuous person was defined as one who observed certain principles and duties[9] or whose behavior was considered admirable by those who observed it.[10]

A further departure from virtue-based ethics occurred in the twentieth century, when the Vienna school of logical positivists turned their attention to ethical discourse. For them, scientific method was the only criterion of true knowledge. They relegated ethics to the same category as theology, myth, or poetry. Ethics became an ineffective enterprise not susceptible to rational analysis. Ethics took on the qualities of an emotivist activity. In this view, the good is a mere statement of preferences. The idea of a virtuous person lost all relationship to any definable good for a given person.

Anglo-American ethics responded to this challenge by taking a severely analytical turn, emphasizing the meaning of ethical terms and the logic of ethical discourse, and developed what came to be called metaethics. Normative statements were eschewed, since there was too much disagreement on the presuppositions of normative ethics and even on the norms of justification of ethical arguments. Moral analysis replaced moral direction, since there could be no agreement on the good to be held out as a goal for persons or rarely could there be a person held out for emulation. In this way ethics assumed a neutralist stance on the most important issues of the day. Doing this, it lost much of its practical value as a guide for living, and its power to stimulate persons toward higher achievements of the good.

This was the situation two decades ago when a remarkable renaissance of interest in ethics began to manifest itself, first in medicine, then in business, law, government, engineering, and a variety of other fields. It is interesting that the revival of interest in ethics should occur in practical endeavors, which require that practical problems be solved in concrete instances. This was especially true in medicine, where technology, social and political events, and the increasingly explicit moral pluralism of contemporary society offered new problems that had not been encountered before.

Traditionally, medical ethics consisted largely of moral aphorisms asserted rather than argued. Most especially absent were the analytical skills then gaining dominance in general ethics. Medicine's own history was part of the history of virtue ethics—what was expected would be done by the good physician as defined in the Hippocratic moral code and its subsequent emendations and enrichment, notably by Stoicism, Christianity, theology, and philosophy.[11] It was shaped further in the Anglo-American ethical movement by the ethos of the gentleman physician as portrayed by Thomas Percival,[12] the Gregories—John and James, father and son—Percival's contemporaries in England, as well as Benjamin Rush and Samuel Bard in America.

In the mid-1960s, for the first time, professional philosophers turned their attention seriously to medical ethics. Surprisingly, except for Plato and Aristotle, this is a subject professional philosophers had neglected as a field of formal and legitimate inquiry. Even in Plato and Aristotle, medicine provided examples and analogies for philosophical reflection, but they were not the subject of formal treatises. The philosophers entered this virgin territory at a critical time, when medicine stood in need of rigorous discourse and analysis if it was not to go the emotivist route. Logical positivism, consciously or not, was the dominant philosophy of medical scientists and medical education. But logical positivism was of little use in medical ethics, since it really denied ethics as a rational discipline and eroded professional ethics as well.

Medical ethicists turned energetically to the seventeenth- and eighteenth-century ethics of Hume, Kant, Mill, and (to a lesser extent) Hutcheson and others in order to address the ethical issues emerging from medical progress in the middle and late 1960s. They turned to prima facie principles that ought to be honored by everyone—namely, respect for persons, beneficence and nonmaleficence, and justice. Some of these early medical ethicists were deontologists; others, utilitarian; some, religious; others, secular. Each set about to unravel the quandaries modern medicine posed in such rich profusion.

The philosophical ethicists achieved considerable success. They rapidly displaced the small cadre of religiously inspired ethicists who had held the field rather loosely, to be sure, for the preceding decade or so. These "theological" ethicists were mostly hospital-oriented pastoral counsellors or chaplains on medical-school campuses. Many were well motivated and helpful in pointing to neglected areas of ethical concern in medical care. But they lacked formal ethical training or had only the minimal training customary in seminary education. This led to an almost exclusive reliance on religious teaching to justify normative statements. In general, they propounded sectarian concerns, each reflecting his or her religious tradition in clinical situations or in the classroom. They were unconvincing to those who did not share their theological presuppositions. These religious ethicists were suspect to many medical personnel, some of whom were nonbelievers and others of whom preferred to separate their medical from their religious commitments. Paradoxically, however, it is this group that opened the discourse on medical campuses and prepared the way for the entry of the philosophical ethicists.[13]

Obvious exceptions to this rule were theologians such as Paul Ramsey, James Gustafson, Joseph Fletcher, Richard McCormick, and William F. May, who began a more rigorous examination of the issues in medical ethics during the late 1960s and some of whom continue their work into the present.[14] In many instances, their work reflected a synthesis of religious thinking about medical concerns during the previous one hundred years. While never abandoning their own religious traditions, these theologians contributed to the emergence of modern medical ethics by providing principles, distinctions, and modes of analysis that are now accepted secular tools of the trade. One did not have to accept their religious convictions, rarely in any event enunciated in the analyses, to grapple with the ideas presented.

Ironically, even at this early stage, resistance to principle-based ethics began to emerge. Joseph Fletcher proposed his "situation ethics" in the late 1950s, in part as a counter to the excessively principle-based ethics of theologians and philosophers after the Second World War.[15] A good example is the thinking of Ramsey, who argued mostly as a deontologist, deductively from principles.[16] A famous debate between Ramsey and McCormick in the 1970s about the use of children in biomedical research exemplifies not only differences in conviction about social expectations of children but also differences in analysis and methodology.[17] While both based their thinking ultimately in the Christian tradition, they differed in the way in which they argued philosophically. William Spurrier's first book attempted to integrate the best of the Catholic and Protestant natural-law traditions.[18]

As experience in the clinical setting expanded, the complexity of issues and individual cases became more manifest. By virtue of their skills in analytical reasoning, these formally trained philosophical ethicists brought analytical rigor, some degree of impartiality, and a willingness to tackle concrete problems—all requirements for a hearing in the medical arena. Those who were successful learned medical terminology and respected the structures of medical authority and the complexity of ethical decision making. They made themselves available for teaching and consultation. They were able to criticize the traditions of medieval ethics and even gain a sympathetic hearing, at least from some physicians.

As a result, contemporary philosophers reshaped the 2,500-year-old tradition of medical ethics in several ways. First, they brought about a transformation in the nature of medical ethics. For the greatest part of its history, medical ethics was essentially a system of morality—a series of deeply held beliefs about the right and the good and the norms of medical behavior. For the first time, medical morality became the subject of analysis, justification, and argumentation. It assumed the aspect of philosophical ethics and became, in some ways, a special branch of philosophical ethics. Second, they transformed medical ethics into a problem-solving enterprise closely akin to clinical problem solving. Medical ethics thus became quandary ethics, almost paradigmatically so. The context of medical ethics focused on the changing sociopolitical, economic, and scientific context of medicine. The complex and unprecedented quandaries demanded practical resolutions for which an analytical framework proved useful. Third, philosophers opened up the field of clinical bioethics to cover ethical decision making at the bedside and to include empirical studies into the process of decision making. This gave new life to descriptive as well as analytical ethics. Fourth, ethical sensitivities, ethical discussions, and ethics committees were encouraged to a degree unheard of in the history of medicine. Finally, philosophical ethicists had a powerful influence in public committees and commissions (such as the President's Commission), in the Congress, in framing legislation, and even in the courts.

The result is that the public and the profession today are attuned to ethics as primarily a problem-solving skill, capable of helping us to make difficult moral choices. This fits well with the individualistic temperament of the times and its moral heterogeneity. The overall effect has been salubrious, especially in confronting the dilemmas of bioethics—the ethic of the applications of the knowledge of biology to human affairs, clinical and otherwise.

But quandary ethics is less successful in the more ancient branch of medical ethics—the ethics of character and the right and proper conduct of the physician as physician. Quandary ethics as it is now practiced places emphasis largely on the process of decision making, on the way to resolve clashes between prima facie principles such as autonomy, beneficence, and justice. It is less successful in recognizing that all choices—those made by the physician, the patient, patient surrogates, or the courts—ultimately must channel through physicians, patients, nurses, and other health professionals. Long-term consequences and the impact of choices on values, families, and the profession are rarely taken into much account.

This unavoidably being the case, the ethics of character and virtue remains, as it has always been, the central issue in medical as well as in any other form of ethics. Yet this is precisely the part of ethics that has not been cultivated by the analytical focus of so much of contemporary medical ethics. This is a serious defect, considering that in the moments of "clinical truth"—i.e., the many times when the physician must exercise judgment on technical matters with implications for the good of the patient—the patient is forced to trust the physician. No contract, no advance directives, no living will, no court order or ethics committee recommendation can cover all eventualities or anticipate those nuances or modulations of judgment that enter into the surgeon's incisions, the internist's prescriptions, or the psychiatrist's counsels. Patient preferences indeed must be honored. They provide a framework within which the ethics of character and virtue must always play a prominent role. But by itself, patient autonomy may not serve every facet of the patient's good.

Earlier we noted how important the role model is for virtue ethics. Thomas Percival is one example of the virtuous physician.[19] Many other physicians have propounded or lived the good way of life in medicine as well. One thinks of Percival's British contemporaries John and James Gregory, and the Americans Samuel Bard and Worthington Hooker, or (to move to more recent examples) Sir William Osler or Francis Peabody. None of these physicians developed a formal philosophical ethics of medicine, but their stories exemplified virtue in their writings, lives, and behavior as physicians.

Percival is a particularly apt example. His personal and medical life reflected a man of character. His written works flow from an underlying moral philosophy. His "Ethics" is a distillation of this moral philosophy, which has its roots in the soil of virtue ethics—the ethics of Aristotle and Plato; the stories of the Christian tradition, scriptural and modern; and the ethics of the "Gentleman" of the eighteenth century. This mixture of influences affected the first code of the American

Medical Association and still shapes the physician's ethical reflections. Today that ethic is in a state of metamorphosis, and its future is problematic.[20] It was displaced in the past quarter century by principle-based quandary ethics. In the past decade, other alternatives have come to challenge both principle-based and the older professional ethics, such as the revival of casuistry and the new emphasis on caring, experiential, and narrative formulation of the moral life.

THE RETURN TO VIRTUE ETHICS

Prominent among the so-called alternatives to principle-based ethics is the return of virtue-based ethics.[21] Virtue ethics has occupied the interest of virtually every major philosopher since its first formal introduction in Greek philosophy. It was the implicit theory behind the ethics of the ancient Chinese and Indian physicians as well.[22] Its interpretations have since been diverse and even contradictory. Since the Enlightenment, particularly with British empiricist philosophers and Kant, it gradually evolved into a system of principles and rules. Yet considerations of virtue continued to hover over moral philosophy. Today, as some of the shortcomings of contemporary ethical theory become manifest, especially in medical ethics, interest is returning to virtue and character. As Von Wright points out, the idea of virtue today is neither obsolete nor accomplished; instead, it is a topic awaiting renewed attention and fresh development.[23]

The nature of these developments is emerging from the growth of recent literature addressing the perennial questions of virtue ethics.[24] This refurbishment of virtue has as yet not produced any startling departures from the more traditional notions. But it has resulted in considerable clarification of the definition, advantages, and defects of the concept of virtue. The ground is being cleared for the return of virtue, not so much as the sole basis of moral philosophy but as an essential element of any ethical theory related, on the one hand, to principles and duties and, on the other, to the motivation for moral behavior. The establishment of these linkages between virtue, principles, cognition of the right and good, and motivation to do the right and good is a central task of contemporary moral philosophy.

Another way of putting this is that morality concerns both the good of actions or conduct, sometimes called objective morality, and the internal motivations and intentions of the agent(s), sometimes called subjective morality. Principles, rules, guidelines, etc., tend to concern the action in question, its objective moral character. Virtue ethics, by contrast, governs the interior life of the agent(s) who perform(s) the action. The reason both are needed is that right actions done with evil intentions or motives are hollow. Guidelines and rules, unless interiorized, will be broken as expedient. On the other hand, without objective morality, any action, such as killing others or stealing, could be justified on the basis of "good intentions." It is the balance of the two approaches that is so important in today's society and so challenging.

Alasdair MacIntyre highlights salient features of post-World War II moral philosophy against which virtue ethics is a reaction.[25] He first points to the almost exclusive focus on moral rules and how they differ from each other. Second, such rules were seen to be impersonal and universal, binding any rational person in any particular set of circumstances. This had a special appeal to the contemporary predisposition to pluralistic, secular, and personal moral choices.

Because of this focus, emphasis was placed on the right (about which there could be rational agreement), as distinguished from the good (about which debate would be interminable and indeterminable).[26] As MacIntyre says: "What is right is what any rational person may require of any other, what is good is a question about which each individual is and ought to be free to make up his or her mind in his or her own way in accordance with his or her private preferences, provided that in acting upon the view which he or she adopts, he or she does not infringe the freedom of any other individual."[27]

This almost classic description of recent ethics clearly demonstrates why the focus on formal rules departs from the virtues, the former dealing with rational criteria for public agreement and public moral policy, and the latter dealing with individuals, the good, and a moral community such as medicine. The problem with rational justification is that agreement rests on acceptance of certain presuppositions about the good and about the good life. These cannot be solely matters of social construction or political accommodation. There are pathological social orders, such as that of Nazi Germany, where physicians adopted a political ideology that converted killing the retarded and genocide into societal healing. Without a theory of the good life and the good society, there is no check on political expediency.[28]

If moral rules are to have binding force, they must have such either from a theory of moral law or from the assent of virtuous individuals who choose the rules as part of their self-definition and moral character. Elizabeth Anscombe is justly famous for her argument that moral injunctions derive their force from whatever gives the point and the purpose for obedience to them. Either that is a divine law beyond particular communities or it is the virtue of the individuals.[29] Since today the former is only what MacIntyre calls a residue of an earlier theological view of society, the latter seems the only place to turn. This is the reason MacIntyre proposed that debate in particular communities can lead from a shared life to a consensus about the common good.[30] Despite further elaboration of the importance of the virtues in more recent works, he still holds that such a conception of the common good can be "sufficiently strong as to place constraints upon a rational understanding of the virtues. It will be in terms of the concrete agreements of social life and the debates which arise from these, and not in the theoretical debates of academic philosophers, that in the end any particular account of the virtues will have to succeed or fail."[31]

One legacy of our own philosophy of medicine is the argument that medicine constitutes a moral community in which the debate about the common good MacIntyre describes could take place, and that an account of the virtues is required therein.

There is as little agreement among virtue theorists as there is among rights and rules theorists. In fact, as MacIntyre's 1988 Gifford Lectures demonstrate, there are at least three modern forms of moral enquiry in which moral debates occur and between which moral conflicts arise. Not only are the differences among different moral enquiries vast and irreconcilable. So, too, are many of the debates among adherents within such systems as Aristotelian and deontological ethics, Nietzschean geneology, or the moral analysis in papal encyclicals. MacIntyre observes that there are fundamentally opposed points of view that lead to inconclusive ethics, since for the warring parties their basic principles seem irrefutable as often do their terms and standards of argument. This has occurred within the discipline of secular humanism as well, ironically, since it was established to correct a kind of moralistic posturing that occurred in religious ethics when an argument did not seem persuasive to opponents.[32] Indeed, the very restoration of virtue ethics itself must address the objection that behind virtue ethics is a kind of dogmatic moralism and is, as Professor Harry Kuitert in the Netherlands has avowed, accompanied by an essential corollary of intolerance.[33]

We think that MacIntyre's description of irreconcilable moral enquiries, while accurate and interesting, tends to overemphasize differences rather than the unifying features of human character and the moral life. To be sure, there are disagreements in principle, in method, in the weight given to history and tradition, and in what counts as good arguments. But within those differences, people may behave similarly with respect to compassion for others, keeping promises, being courageous, and acting prudently. The virtues, therefore, as elements of character, may transcend differences in modes of moral enquiry because they are ultimately related to what it is to be fully human. The effort to seek a morality grounded in our common humanity should not be abandoned, notwithstanding the current incommensurability of notions of the good. In any case, we believe that in the limited case of medicine, it is easier to find agreement on the good, on ends, and on purposes.[34]

THE THEOLOGICAL VIRTUES

Christian ethics, like secular ethics, relies on a combination of principles, rules, and virtues. In the Christian worldview, much emphasis is placed on the kind of person one ought to be, on conversion of one's way of life to bring it closer to the way of life Jesus manifested in the Gospels. Indeed, it is from the example of Jesus' life and his teachings that the whole of Christian ethics takes its inspiration and justification. The virtues inherent in the Sermon on the Mount are the virtues by which Christians are expected ultimately to live and shape their own lives.

In Catholic moral theology since the late Middle Ages, casuistry as a method of assessing guilt during aural confession took a dominant role, sometimes overshadowing the primacy of personal character and virtue. The inspiration for Catholic medical morality, however, was always the message of the Gospels and the virtues of faith, hope, and charity—which are called the supernatural, or theological, virtues. These, with the four cardinal virtues (prudence, temperance, fortitude, and justice), constituted the substance of what may be termed Christian virtue ethics.

Christian virtue ethics evolved over the centuries as a result of the confrontation by the early church fathers and doctors of Christianity with the philosophical heritage of the Greco-Roman world. Their commitment to faith in a source of morality transcending humanity presented a question of the most serious proportions: how were they to reconcile their religious faith with the reasoned arguments of the pagan philosophers? Meeting the challenge was crucial to the construction of a Christian ethic, one that did not defy reason yet was faithful to the revealed truths of the Jewish and Christian Bibles.

Two Christian teachers are preeminent in the effort to reconcile pagan and secular philosophy with Christian revelation—St. Augustine and St. Thomas. For our purposes, it is essential to confine our comments on their extensive work on faith and reason to the question of virtue as it was received from Greco-Roman philosophy. Each accepted the central idea of virtues as traits of character, as perfections of human conduct of a moral and intellectual kind. Both incorporated the classic cardinal virtues into their moral philosophies. Both also saw the insufficiency of the natural virtues in living the fullness of the Christian life.

Of the two, Augustine's effort was the more complex, in large measure because it comprised his own spiritual autobiography. As Augustine went from paganism through conversion to Christianity, his concept of virtue changed accordingly. He began with Cicero's rendition of the Stoic philosophy, according to which happiness, virtue, and self-determination are convergent. As his faith commitment grew, Augustine realized that knowledge of the good is not sufficient for the good life and that motivation of the will is necessary if good is to be chosen over evil. To motivate the will, some transcendent good is necessary. Augustine found this in the Neoplatonists. In his conversion to Christian belief, Augustine realized that this transcendent good is a Supreme God who illumines the world and human intelligence by grace and thus motivates it to do the good: "And this is truly perfect virtue—reason arriving at its end after which the blessed life follows."[35]

Augustine examined the claims of both the Peripatetics and the Stoics that virtue will lead to happiness in this life even in the face of grave hardship. He criticized their concept of virtue for not appreciating that happiness is unattainable when the end is only natural good; happiness requires pursuit of the eternal good, and that good comes only through faith, hope, and charity, the virtues through which God illumines the human will and intellect and ordains them to their proper end in God:[36] "Genuine virtues can exist only in those who are endowed with true piety. . . . [Genuine virtues] . . . do say that our human life, though it is compelled by all the great evils of this age to be wretched, is happy in the expectation of a future life insofar as it enjoys the expectation of salvation, too."[37]

In the *Confessions*, Augustine explored the complexity of moral psychology in the way the affections can influence the virtues. Augustine's version of the virtues, therefore, combined a cognitive component (i.e., a proper vision of the good) with an affective component (i.e., the conformation of desire with a vision of the good).[38] The supreme good draws persons forward. In the end, will takes precedence over intellect, but the will must be directed and shaped by humility.

Augustine defined virtue in several different places and in somewhat different ways, for example, "The function of virtue is the good use of things of which we can also make a bad use"[39] and "For virtue makes both good use of the self and the other good things that go to make a man happy."[40] Gilson points to Augustine's definition of virtue in *De civitate Dei*, "Ordo est amoris," which Gilson renders as "Love's submission to order."[41]

For Augustine, as it was for Aquinas, charity is the ordering virtue of the Christian life, the source of resolution of internal conflict as well as the rectification of the passions, directing them to their proper ends. All the other virtues are reduced to, and are subservient to, this virtue of charity, i.e., "the licit love of man for man, love of man for God, love of God for man."[42] In this sense, Augustine held to the unity of the virtues—the natural with the supernatural. Augustine agreed with the pagan philosophers that virtue resides in a "wisely conducted life" but "this is not enough, to live rightly takes on a new meaning if we have faith which enables us to love rightly which is to attain eternal life."[43] It is the "stupid pride" of the Stoics and the "surprising error" of the Peripatetics to suppose that the supreme good is to be found in this life and that they can be "the agents of their own happiness."[44]

Augustine's concept of virtue was a complex amalgam of pagan philosophy and Christian theology. Its definition evolved throughout his life as he grew in his perceptions of divine grace and its place in human willing. Thomas Aquinas, on the other hand, began his study of both philosophy and theology as a committed Christian. He had access to the full text of Aristotle's *Nicomachean Ethics*, which became available in part (books 2 and 3) in the late twelfth century and in full in the early thirteenth century.[45] Thomas developed the concept of virtue as conceived in Aristotle and Augustine, and he amended each. The broad outline of his conception of natural virtue follows the essential elements of Aristotle's—virtue as a character trait, as a teleological *habitus*, something learned by practice and guided by practical reason.

Like Aristotle, Aquinas interpreted the natural virtues as inclinations to the good, to what makes a man good and his work according to reason. Virtue is something within human nature that inclines us to those acts which fulfill our nature as human beings. Thus, like Aristotle, Aquinas taught a teleological theory of the virtues, seeing them as dispositions or excellences of character that perfect our capacity to lead fully human lives. Aquinas accepted the classical list of cardinal virtues, i.e., temperance, fortitude, justice, and wisdom, as they had been enunciated in Plato.[46] He saw Plato's version of wisdom as practical wisdom—-the chief of the natural virtues, the ordering virtue that enables us to discern what is the right thing to do in the complexity of concrete situations. This power of discernment is prudence, the chief of the natural virtues, which Aquinas described as *recta ratio agibilium*—a rightness in acting according to reason. Aquinas' prudence is akin to Aristotle's *phronēsis*, or practical wisdom.

Also like Aristotle, Aquinas held that the virtues are ascertainable by human reason and perfected by training and practice. "Fitness as for virtue is in us by nature but the fullness of virtue comes by practice."[47] Thus, Aquinas' answer to Meno's question "Is virtue something that can be taught?"[48] is in the affirmative.

But like Augustine, Thomas pointed out the insufficiency of the natural virtues for full human happiness and so complemented Aristotle's natural virtues with the supernatural virtues. These are not simply extensions of the natural virtues. They are, as Sokolowski puts it, "specifically the dispositions for acting in the setting disclosed by Christian faith; they are the sources of the reaction we are to have to the God Who creates without any need for creation and Who involves us in His own life through His Son. And, strictly speaking, we simply cannot act on our own in this new setting."[49]

Aristotle's and Plato's conception of virtue was based in the nature of the human person as they saw it, unenlightened by the revelations of the Jewish and Christian Scriptures. This conception was necessarily insufficient for Augustine and Aquinas. As committed Christians, they subscribed to a theological anthropology that held the ultimate end of human existence to be beatific union with the Triune God. Their views of the relationship of the natural moral virtues to Christian belief differed, however. Augustine reduced all the virtues, natural and supernatural, to charity. Aquinas maintained the integrity of the natural virtues, even for the person who accepts the Gospels and their doctrine of salvation. As Sokolowski puts it, "What is good by nature remains good in the setting in which grace is required; its goodness is in fact enhanced not distorted by the new context."[50] This is another way of stating the familiar Thomistic precept that faith perfects nature; it does not destroy or replace it.

The supernatural virtues are faith, hope, and charity, and we shall examine each of these separately insofar as they indicate the virtues the Christian physician should exhibit in his or her healing activity. For a more general point of view, we may regard the theological virtues as those which dispose the Christian to the supernatural good of human nature—to its destination of salvation and union with God.

Several recent treatises by Christian theologians, philosophers, and others have examined in some detail the way Christian belief modifies the exercise of the natural virtues and the way the natural and supernatural virtues differ from each other.[51] For our purposes, it suffices to outline some of the ways in which the theological virtues differ from the natural and interact with each other.

For one thing, the supernatural virtues are not acquired by human effort or actions. They are freely given gifts of God. They are infused in us by God[52] and possessed by humans through grace. They dispose us to perfect our lives with respect to our spiritual destiny and, thus, in our life with God. The theological virtues are ordered to our true spiritual end, while the natural virtues are ordered to our natural ends in human affairs. In this sense, the theological virtues are primary and the natural virtues are virtues in a derived or secondary sense.[53]

From a theological or supernatural perspective, sin is not simply vice, or the lack of virtue. It is an offense against the Creator, and destroys grace. Since the infused virtues come through grace, they, too, are lost by sin. With proper repentance, grace is restored, and with it, the possibility of infused virtue is restored as well.[54] Thus, sin has a deeper significance, since it involves loss of the true end of human life, while vice distorts attainment of only the natural fulfillment or happiness of the vicious person.

The theological virtues do not destroy the natural virtues or divide human life into two discrete spheres of action. Rather, the Christian viewpoint confirms "what is good by nature and [appreciates] that what is good according to nature is not simply good in itself but also good because created and therefore willed by God."[55] It is faith in the goodness of God and creation, together with hope of one's salvation and that of one's fellows, that shapes all the natural inclinations to the good that the natural virtues bring to human action.

Through the supernatural virtues, the natural virtues are elevated to the level of grace, i.e., to a degree of perfection inappreciable without them. Humility, solicitude for the poor, patience, suffering, and temperance are transmuted into acts of charity and thereby strengthened and expanded. For Plato and Aristotle, the virtues were natural excellences (*aretai*). But the theological virtues are excellences in the spiritual life, and that takes ethics beyond itself. We may speak of virtue theory with respect to the natural virtues, but the Beatitudes are not formulae for abstract good but, as Guardini called them, a "whole new existence."[56]

The introduction of the supernatural virtues into virtue theory by Aquinas opened the question of their relationship with the natural virtues. This is an issue that was not clearly or directly set out in Augustine, where the emphasis on grace sometimes seems to overshadow the worthiness of the natural virtues.

The relationship between the natural and supernatural virtues is complex in Aquinas.[57] Clearly the natural virtues are not sufficient for salvation, yet they are not obliterated by the supernatural virtues. The natural virtues remain requisite for our actions in the world, but we need the supernatural virtues for our actions in the setting of Christian belief. We cannot attain the supernatural virtues by our own efforts, while we can attain some significant measure of the natural virtues.

On Sokolowski's reading of Aquinas,[58] a further distinction exists between the acquired natural moral virtues and the infused moral virtues. They are different in species in that the infused moral virtues more specifically dispose to perfection of our life with God, so that prudence, temperance, or fortitude are ordained to our ultimate end, rather than simply to fulfillment of our natural ends in life. The infused moral virtues do not impose obligations at odds with nature. They confirm that what is good by nature is good because created and willed by God. "What is good by nature is not set over against what is good by grace but is integrated into it."[59]

We shall have occasion in the chapters that follow to see how the theological virtues ordain for the Christian physician a way of life and indicate the kind of person she/he should be and the kind of life in medicine she/he should live. None of this abolishes or engulfs the natural virtues of medicine but takes them to levels of perfection beyond ethics in the ordinary sense.

PRINCIPLES AND THE VIRTUES, NATURAL AND THEOLOGICAL

The dominant approach to biomedical ethical problems today is through application of the four prima facie principles of justice, autonomy, beneficence, and nonmaleficence. Much of the progress made in recent years may be attributed to the creative application of these principles. As the gradual inclusion of this method became widespread in medical and clinical ethics, the limitations of prima facie principles were manifest in the nuances and complexities of ethical decision making at the bedside. As we noted earlier, a backlash against "principlism" has begun to set in.[60] Critics have pointed to the abstract nature of principles, their failure to capture the richness and complexity of the moral life, and their rigidity. This has led to the search for alternative ways of doing ethics. Some have turned to an ethics more immersed in the concrete details of the personal and emotional lives of those affected by the decision. For some this turn away from principles leads to hermeneutics,[61] and for others to an ethics of story.[62]

Warren Reich, for example, has appealed to ethicists to analyze cases involving defective newborns from a richer perspective he calls an experiential ethic.[63] As we understand him, this is not virtue ethic per se but something bordering on psychologically attentive ethics. Nonetheless, this point is a good example of an analysis of an extremely difficult case that embodies other factors than one in which rationalism alone prevails. But herein lies the difficulty of alternatives to principles.

Appeals to experience, even appeals to virtue alone, will always be insufficient. Our experience might be limited. We may become overwhelmed by the emotional content of the decisions to be made. Experience constantly changes. Tomorrow's decision may not resemble today's. The number and background of the persons making the decisions also vary and will affect the nature of the decision. Similarly, an appeal to trust in the virtues of the caregiver or medical researcher admits of too much risk and variability in what the moral agent takes to be a virtue. Most consider virtue ethic a poor substitute for serious social and public policy, where there is no single moral agent but a collective effort in which compromise, and not excellence of intent or action, is primary.

Turning away from principles to experience bears a relationship to virtue-based ethics, since virtue-based ethics also recognizes the central importance of the character of the agent in moral decisions and acts. After all, principles are selected and interpreted by persons. They must be weighed against other alternatives, conflicts among them resolved, and underlying values asserted or denied. This is a complex moral task. The gap between perception of the right and good and doing the right and good thing is wider for some people than for others. The character of the agent and his or her moral psychology are the filters through which prima facie principles are reflected or refracted. Thus, the inseparability of the agent from the principles employed in an act poses a large and still problematic conceptual problem—how are principle and virtue (or the other alternative forms of ethics) to be linked?

Virtue ethics is not a salvation theme for the difficulties of principle-based ethics. It has its limitations as well. The definition of the good person is variable in a morally pluralistic society; there is a tendency toward subjectivism in defining virtues and vices; there is a corresponding vagueness in the absence of specific action guidelines; role models may differ over time. Clearly the strengths and weaknesses of a principle-based ethical system and a virtue-based system balance each other. A complete moral philosophy must take each into account. This is especially true of a philosophy of medicine and medical ethics.

The question is important for the relationship of the theological virtues to principles. This is not the place to examine how faith, hope, and charity link, for example, with the well-established principles of Catholic moral theology—the principle of double effect, of formal and material cooperation, of integrity of the whole, of proportionality, etc. But to effect this link is a necessary effort for Catholic medical ethics. Just as the theological virtues modify and perfect the natural virtues, they modify and perfect the principles of Catholic moral philosophy and theology. This linkage is yet to be fully forged, since it brings together the casuistic tradition, which has been dominant in Catholic moral theology, with the newer emphasis on virtues, which has received less recent attention in that tradition.

Finally, a word is in order on how the theological virtues would change the way medical ethics is construed and practiced. In a sense, this is the major enterprise of the rest of this book. For the moment at least, we can say that the theological virtues will affect what it is to be a physician and the way the popular four-principle approach and the virtues internal to medicine are used in making ethical decisions. For a physician committed to the Christian ethic, each principle and each virtue is raised to the level of grace. Beneficence, for example, goes far beyond nonmaleficence to embrace doing good for others even when it involves significant effacement of self-interest, and it arises from a disinterested motive of love for neighbor. Autonomy becomes more than a negative prerogative; it becomes a positive respect for the enormous dignity of the patient as a child of God who has autonomy because of God-given dignity. Humans have dignity not because they are autonomous but because they are humans. Justice becomes charitable justice not by the strict weighing of what is owed by rule of law but by the rule of charity.

The remainder of this book examines the ways the theological virtues reshape both the natural virtues and the philosophical principles on which clinical ethical decisions are made.

CONCLUSION

As can be seen from our sketch of virtue theory in a companion work,[64] an enormous amount of development in virtue theory itself, as well as ethical theory in general, has taken place. Only in the last few years has a resurgence of interest in virtue theory occurred. Now attention is focused in medical ethics on how to link principles, norms, and axioms with clinical casuistry, which is so much a part of medical practice. It seems obvious that, despite a proliferation of policies and guidelines, the individual physician, along with the patient, must be habitually disposed toward the good and generally to be trusted with this habituation. Terrible incidents can occur in medicine and medical practice, from outright fraud to direct harm to patients, incidents that casuistry and syllogistic deduction cannot, by themselves, avoid. Our exploration of the link between the virtues and the qualities necessary for medical practice starts with the central virtues of faith, hope and healing, and charity in the next chapters. First we explore Christian virtue theory in more detail in the next chapter.

NOTES

1. Edmund D. Pellegrino and David C. Thomasma, *The Virtues in Medical Practice* (New York: Oxford University Press, 1993).

2. Catholic Church, *Catechism of the Catholic Church* (Mahwah, N.J.: Paulist Press, 1994), n. 1834, p. 451.

3. Servais Pinckaers, "Les sources de la morale chrétien: Sa méthode, son contenu, son histoire," in *Études D'Éthique Chrétienne*, 2d ed. (Freibourg Suiss: Éditions Universitaires, 1990).

4. Catholic Church, *Universal Catechism*, n. 1840, p. 451.

5. Plato, "Meno" and "Protagoras" in *Plato: The Collected Dialogues* ed. Edith Hamilton and Huntington Cairns (Princeton: Princeton University Press, 1985), pp. 353–384 and 308–352 respectively.

6. Aristotle, "Nicomachean Ethics," in *The Basic Works of Artistotle*, ed. Richard McKeon (New York: Random House, 1941), 1105b: 25–26, p. 957.

7. Aristotle, "Nicomachean Ethics," 1106a: 16–17, p. 957.

8. Aristotle, "Nicomachean Ethics," 1106a: 22–24, p. 957.

9. Immanuel Kant, "Metaphysical Principles of Virtue (Part II of The Metaphysics of Morals)," in *Ethical Philosophy*, trans. James W. Ellington (Indianapolis, Ind.: Hackett Publishing Company, 1983), pp. 31ff.

10. David Hume, *Enquiries Concerning Human Understanding and the Principles of Morals*, ed. L. A. Selby-Biggs (Oxford: Clarendon Press, 1980).

11. Pedro Lain Entralgo, *Doctor and Patient*, trans. Frances Partridge (New York: McGraw-Hill, 1969).

12. Edmund D. Pellegrino, "Percival's Medical Ethics: The Moral Philosophy of an 18th-Century English Gentleman," *Archives of Internal Medicine* 146 (November 1986): 2265–2269.

13. Edmund D. Pellegrino and Thomas A. McElhinny, *Teaching Ethics, the Humanities, and Human Values in Medical Schools: A Ten Year Overview* (Washington, D.C.: Institute on Human Values in Medicine of the Society for Health and Human Values, 1982).

14. Paul Ramsey, *The Patient as Person: Explorations in Medical Ethics* (New Haven: Yale University Press, 1970); Joseph Fletcher, *The Ethics of Genetic Control: Ending Reproductive Roulette* (Buffalo: Prometheus Books, 1988); William F. May, *The Physician's Covenant: Images of the Healer in Medical Ethics* (Philadelphia: Westminster Press, 1983); Richard McCormick, *The Critical Calling: Reflections of Moral Dilemmas Since Vatican II* (Washington, D.C.: Georgetown University Press, 1989).

15. Joseph Fletcher, *Situation Ethics: The New Morality* (Philadelphia: Westminster Press, 1966).

16. Ramsey, *Patient as Person*.

17. Glenn C. Graber and David C. Thomasma, *Theory and Practice in Medical Ethics* (New York: Continuum, 1989).

18. William A. Spurrier, *Natural Law and the Ethics of Love* (Philadelphia: Westminster Press, 1974).

19. Thomas Percival, *Medical Ethics, or a Code of Institutions and Precepts Adapted to The Professional Conduct of Physicians and Surgeons* [reprinted from the 1805 version] (Birmingham, Ala.: Classics of Medicine Library, 1985).

20. Edmund D. Pellegrino, "Foreword: Thomas Percival, The Ethics Beneath the Etiquette," in Percival, *Medical Ethics*, pp. 1–65.

21. Alternatives are discussed in Pellegrino and Thomasma, *Virtues in Medical Practice*.

22. Cf. Sreedhara Menon, "Oath of Initiation (from the *Caraka Samhita*)," *Medical History* 14 (1970): 295–296; Chen Shih-kung, "Five Commandments and Ten Requirements of Physicians," trans. Tao Lee, *Bulletin of the History of Medicine* 13 (1943): 271–272; and O. Jaggi, "History of Medical Ethics: India,"

in *Encyclopedia of Bioethics* (Vol. III), ed. Warren T. Reich (New York: The Free Press, 1978), pp. 906–911.

23. Georg H. Von Wright, *The Varieties of Goodness* (New York: Humanities Press, Routledge and Keagan Paul, 1963).

24. Alasdair MacIntyre, *After Virtue: A Study in Moral Theory* (Notre Dame, Ind.: University of Notre Dame Press, 1984); Michael Slote, *From Morality to Virtue* (New York: Oxford University Press, 1992); Elizabeth Anscombe, *Collected Papers: Ethics, Religion and Politics* (Minneapolis: University of Minnesota Press, 1981); Philippa Foot, *Virtues and Vices* (Oxford: Basil Blackwell, 1978); Edmund L. Pincoffs, *Quandaries and Virtues: Against Reductivism in Ethics* (Lawrence, Kansas: University Press of Kansas, 1986).

25. Alasdair MacIntyre, "The Return to Virtue Ethics," in *The Twenty-Fifth Anniversary of Vatican II: A Look Back and a Look Ahead* [Proceedings of the Ninth Bishops' Workshop, Dallas, TX], ed. Russell Smith (Braintree, Mass.: Pope John Center, 1990), pp. 239–249.

26. Richard M. Hare, *Moral Thinking* (Oxford: Clarendon Press, 1981).

27. MacIntyre, "Return to Virtue Ethics," p. 240.

28. Robert Kruschwitz and Robert C. Roberts, eds., *The Virtues: Contemporary Essays on Moral Character* (Belmont, Cal.: Wadsworth Publishing Company, 1987).

29. Elizabeth Anscombe, "Modern Moral Philosophy," in *Collected Papers*, p. 30.

30. MacIntyre, *After Virtue*. See United States Catholic Conference, National Christian Conference and the Synagogue Council, "The Common Good: Old Idea, New Urgency," *Origins* 23, no. 6 (1993): 82–86.

31. MacIntyre, "Return to Virtue Ethics," p. 248.

32. Alasdair MacIntyre, *Three Rival Versions of Moral Enquiry: Encyclopedia, Genealogy, and Tradition* (Notre Dame, Ind.: University of Notre Dame Press, 1990), p. 7.

33. As noted in Wybo J. Dondorp, *The Rehabilitation of Virtue* [Ph.D. Dissertation] (Amsterdam: Vrije Universiteit, 1994). Dondorp builds on the work of the Dutch theologian and ethicist, G. Brillenburg Wurth, who, as early as 1958, published *Eerherstel van de deugd* in an effort to rehabilitate virtue theory.

34. Pellegrino and Thomasma, *Virtues in Medical Practice*.

35. St. Augustine, *Soliloquies*, trans. Thomas F. Gilligan (New York: Cima Publishing Company, 1948), p. 360.

36. St. Augustine, "The City of God," in *The Basic Writings of St. Augustine* (New York, NY: Random House, 1948), Book XIX, p. iv.

37. Augustine, "City of God," p. 94.

38. James Wetzel, *Augustine and the Limits of Virtue* (New York: Cambridge University Press, 1992), pp. 14–15.

39. St. Augustine, "Retractions," in *Philosophy in the Middle Ages: The Christian, Islamic, and Jewish Traditions*, ed. Arthur Hyman and James J. Walsh (Indianapolis, Ind.: Hackett Publishing Company, 1973), p. 66.

40. Augustine, *Soliloquies*, p. 360.

41. Étienne Gilson, *The Christian Philosophy of St. Augustine* (New York: Random House, 1960), p. 166.

42. Augustine, "City of God," Bk. XV, Ch. 22, p. 307.

43. Augustine, "City of God," Bk. XIX, Ch.III.

44. Augustine, "City of God," Bk. XIX, Ch. IV.

45. Scott MacDonald, "Later Medieval Ethics," in *A History of Western Ethics*, ed. Lawrence Becker and Charlotte Becker (New York: Garland Publishing Company, 1992), p. 54.

46. Plato, "The Republic," in *Plato: The Collected Dialogues*, ed. Edith Hamilton and Huntington Cairns (Princeton: Princeton University Press, 1985), 4:427e, p. 669; and *Wisdom* 8:7.

47. St. Thomas Aquinas, *Summa Theologiae* [Vol.32] trans. and ed. Thomas Gilby (New York: Blackfriars, 1966) II-II, q. 108, a. 2, p. 121.

48. Plato, "Meno," in *Plato: The Collected Dialogues*, 70a, p. 354.

49. Robert Sokolowski, *The God of Faith and Reason* (Notre Dame, Ind.: University of Notre Dame Press, 1982), p. 72.

50. Sokolowski, *God of Faith and Reason*, p. 70.

51. Yves Simon, *The Definition of Moral Virtue*, ed. Vukan Kuic (New York: Fordham University Press, 1986); Romano Cessario, *The Moral Virtues and Theological Ethics* (Notre Dame, Ind.: University of Notre Dame Press, 1991); Jean Porter, *The Recovery of Virtue: The Relevance of Aquinas for Christian Ethics* (Louisville, Kentucky: Westminster/John Knox Press, 1990).

52. Aquinas, *Summa Theologiae* [Vol. 23], I-II, q. 65, art. 3, pp. 186–190 and [Vol. 5] I, q. 19, a. 7, pp. 30-34.

53. Sokolowski, *God of Faith and Reason*, p. 70.

54. Aquinas, *Summa Theologiae* [Vol. 23], I-II, q. 65, art. 3, pp. 186–190 and [Vol. 5] I, q. 19, a. 7, pp. 30–34.

55. Sokolowski, *God of Faith and Reason*, p. 83.

56. Roman Guardini, *The Lord* (Chicago, Ill.: Regnery Press, 1954), p. 79.

57. Sokolowski, *God of Faith and Reason*, pp. 76–87.

58. Sokolowski, *God of Faith and Reason*, p. 70 (referring to St. Thomas Aquinas, *Summa Theologiae* [Vol. 23], I-II, q. 65, a. 2, pp. 184–87 and q. 63, a. 3, pp. 158–61).

59. Sokolowski, *God of Faith and Reason*, p. 83.

60. K. Danner Clouser and Bernard Gert, "A Critique of Principlism," *Journal of Medicine and Philosophy* 15, no. 2 (1990): 219–36.

61. See *Theoretical Medicine* 15, no. 4 (1994).

62. Kathryn M. Hunter, *Doctors' Stories: The Narrative Structure of Medical Knowledge* (Princeton: Princeton University Press, 1991).

63. Warren T. Reich, "Caring for Life in the First of It: Moral Paradigms for Perinatal and Neonatal Ethics," *Seminars in Perinatology* 11, no. 3 (1987): 279–87.

64. Pellegrino and Thomasma, *Virtues in Medical Practice*, pp. 3–17.

2

Christian Virtue Ethics

A Christian perspective on morals—medical or otherwise—implies a coherent view of the moral life that transcends purely philosophical ethics in distinctive ways. What these ways consist in, whether they are different in kind or degree, and whether they entail a distinctive moral life are important and problematic questions.

At a minimum, a Christian perspective must encompass fundamental questions: Does a Christian belief entail a content and methodology distinct from, and closed to, philosophical ethics? Are uncritical fideism or unrelenting rationalism the only alternatives? Is ethics as a reasoned discipline reconcilable with ethics as a response to the moral imperatives of the Gospels or their authoritative interpretation by the church?

Many of these issues are engaged throughout this volume and in contemporary theological discourse. They form the inescapable backdrop for this chapter, which examines them in the limited confines of professional ethics. They are especially pertinent in any consideration of charity, the central virtue of the Christian life. It is the virtue of charity that above all shapes the whole of Christian medical morals, as it does every other aspect of the moral life.

This chapter examines some of the conceptual relationships between reason and charity in traditional and contemporary ethical discourse. Two important caveats must be established at the outset.

First, the Christian virtue of charity is the central distinguishing feature of a Catholic and Christian perspective on the moral life. Christian ethics is by definition, therefore, an "agapeistic" ethics. But this is not synonymous with the situation ethics of Joseph Fletcher, which also claims to be agapeistic.[1] Fletcher's form of ethics eschews principle and precept. It dissociates reason and charity in ways incompatible with a Catholic perspective. A situational ethics is by definition antithetical to the Catholic tradition in ethics because it does not relate the situation to the virtue of the individual and to moral principles that cannot be violated.

A second caveat is that an agapeistic ethics does not necessarily place orthopraxy and orthodoxy in opposition to each other.[2] Rather, it advances the special task of Catholic and Christian ethics to reconcile doctrine and practice in a harmonious equilibrium. In that equilibrium the moral life of the Catholic Christian becomes the integrated whole that both reason and faith require.

Three themes run through this book. First, any comprehensive Christian medical moral philosophy ought to be grounded in the nature of medicine itself as a human activity. On grounds of natural reason alone, the nature of medical activity imposes certain specific obligations on the physician and other health professionals. This is the "internal" morality of medicine itself, a morality fitted to the ends of the kind of activity that medical activity is.[3]

Second, a Christian perspective begins, but does not end, with this internal morality, which by itself is insufficient. This intense morality lacks dimensions of insight and obligation that grow out of Christian teachings. Charity thus informs ethical reasoning in certain specific ways. Just how charity and reason relate is a central question for traditional and contemporary accounts of the moral life. A religious perspective for our times should try to reconcile the traditional and the contemporary views.

Third, though the relationships between reason and charity and between traditional and contemporary views of Christian ethics are still under discussion, certain practical moral choices are clearly more consistent with the virtue of charity than others. These choices are made differently than is normally the case if one professes to be a Christian as well as a physician, nurse, or administrator.

Several topics highly relevant to the Catholic perspective are consciously excluded in this book. First is the relationship between ethics as a discipline and the teaching authority of the official magisterium. This subject has been definitively set forth in the recent encyclical *Veritatis Splendor.*[4] Second is the place of the casuistic method in moral decision making. This method has enjoyed a recent revival.[5] It is, however, no longer peculiar to Catholic moral theology, and in any case, we regard it as a heuristic aid, not as a source of normative ethics. Third is the whole range of specific moral questions relating to human life, reproduction, sexuality, abortion, assisted suicide, etc. These are the subjects of several good texts and a plethora of articles of recent date.[6]

Our focus will be primarily on virtue ethics, on the moral *agent* rather than the *act*, the *circumstances*, or the *consequences*. We will focus on the kind of person a Catholic physician, nurse, or other health professional ought to be. Although our emphasis is on virtue-based ethics, we recognize the need to link virtue theory to principles, rules, and duties for any comprehensive theory of the Catholic Christian moral life.[7]

THE INTERNAL MORALITY OF MEDICINE

Many contemporary thinkers conclude that belief in God, Creation, Redemption, and the Incarnation does not provide specific answers to general or medical moral problems. They argue that the whole of the right and the good is open to human reason, since the good is intrinsic to the world God created. On this view, God asks obedience to moral law because it is good; moral law is not good simply because God asks obedience to it.

Josef Fuchs summarizes this line of argument as follows: Medicine is a moral enterprise because it deals with human problems. The ethics of medicine derives from medicine as a human activity. Its moral nature is prior to, or at least not dependent upon, faith. Medical ethics, thus, must accord with human understanding, and in this sense it has a certain autonomy.[8] John Langan makes the same point, underscoring the importance of philosophy and scientific data in the development of bioethics.[9]

Robert Sokolowski follows essentially the same line of argument. He begins with the phenomenology of medicine as a special kind of human activity.[10] He focuses on the art of medicine and the way it functions in the physician-patient relationship. What is at stake is the personhood of the patient. The patient and the physician, as rational beings, each play a part in effecting the end of medicine, which is the good of the patient. In this relationship, the physician is the embodiment of the medical art, whose end is the patient's good.

On Sokolowski's view, beneficence is a moral obligation that is programmed into the art. A physician who does harm violates the art. A physician faithful to the art becomes a good moral agent and is ennobled. Thus, the art establishes the way in which physician and patient should relate to each other. This is the "internal" morality of medicine itself, and it is derivable by reason from the nature of medicine as a particular kind of human activity. We have argued similarly for the obligations that are derivable from the fact of illness, the vulnerability of the patient, and the physician's promise to help.[11]

According to Sokolowski, Christian belief affects this internal morality of medicine in several ways. It reveals more fully and truthfully the good intrinsic to the art; it corrects the tendency to reductionism and the neglect of form characteristic of modern scientific medicine; and it highlights the dignity of the human persons—doctor and patient—who confront each other in the healing relationship.

Christian belief thus expands the range of insights available to ethics as a reasoned discipline.[12] As Lisa Cahill points out, the Catholic perspective operates best when it brings together philosophical reflection, religious images, logical interpretation, concrete human experience, and magisterial teachings. Each contributes to a fuller comprehension of the natural law and enables Christians to make moral choices in conformity with the spirit of Gospel teachings.[13]

On this view, ethics as a reasoned discipline becomes insufficient alone to express the whole of the moral life. The virtues themselves must be included.[14] Christian moral life is more than the application of principles and rules. It offers insights from the Gospel teachings on charity that are not admissible into ethical discourse by those who reject those teachings. It should demonstrate commitments through actions.

Romano Guardini, in his meditation on the Sermon on the Mount, argues that a principle-based ethics reduces a way of life to a set of rules. In a whole new existence such as Jesus taught, an ethos is immediately evident. "Only in love is fulfillment of the ethical possible. Love is the New Testament."[15] Thomas Merton concurs: "We must of course point out that mere ethics, as a moral philosophy, has its limitations. It needs to be completed. . . . [It arises] out of the deep personal relation of man to God in saving grace by which man is oriented to his true and perfect finality, his ultimate fulfillment as a person in the love of God and of his fellow man in God."[16]

THE PHILOSOPHICAL STATUS OF A CHARITY-BASED ETHIC

We agree with Guardini and Merton that we must go beyond "mere ethics" to fulfill the Christian commandment of love. Like St. Paul (Colossians 2:8), we must be wary of the possibility of the submergence of charity by philosophy. Both Guardini and Merton recognize that it is the complementarity of faith and reason that distinguishes the Catholic moral tradition and preserves it against the heart-over-head experiential ethics of Jansenists, Quietists, and Modernists. These movements tended to reconcile the emotional and historical life with the intellectual life by retreating from the notion that some permanent or stable principles can guide the moral life as well. Nonetheless, a charity-based agapeistic ethic poses difficult philosophical questions that remain problematic.

William Frankena, for example, notes the philosophical dilemma in the double imperative of Christian ethics—to love God and one's neighbor as oneself.[17] He argues that an agapeistic ethic could be grounded in the principle of love of neighbor but that love of God could not be derived from beneficence alone. Without faith in God's existence we could not derive the command to love God. But for the Christian this is the ground of an agapeistic ethic. The Christian loves God because God has created all that is good. Charitable beneficence is grounded in God's love for us and in his revelation of that love. It follows from faith, which is the "virtue of entry" into the Christian life and which assures us of a personal relationship of love with God.

Yet, Frankena admits that "there is a sense in which the law of love underlies the entire moral law even if this cannot be derived from it."[18] That the law and all the prophets are summed up in the love of God and neighbor is not a conclusion of reason, but neither does it violate reason.

These metaethical difficulties do not preclude the possibility of a Christian moral philosophy. Every moral philosophy rests ultimately on some ordering principle, whether it be the categorical imperative, a principle of utility, moral sentiment, love of man without God, or love of man because of God. In each philosophy there is, at the outset, an act of faith in some ordering principle. To deny that any such principle exists is itself an ordering principle. For the Christian, the existence of God and revelation is one such starting position. It does not, on that account, have a lesser claim to coherence than moral philosophies that deny both God and revelation.

In recent years, Catholic thinkers have approached the question of a specifically Christian and Catholic ethics with renewed interest. They have examined the ways in which charity and reason are related by linking traditional moral theology to contemporary philosophy and psychology. These attempts are not always mutually reconcilable. But they do open up possibilities for the fresh synthesis of old and new ideas that a comprehensive Catholic moral philosophy requires today.

For Catholics, the central question is how to reconcile an ethics based in reason, principles, and precepts with the fact that the fullness of the Christian ethos of charitable love is somehow beyond ethics, in Guardini's and Merton's sense. Is it possible to avoid the extremes of an unthinking, totally experiential fideism on the one hand and a rigid, unfeeling, legalistic rationalism on the other?

Garth Hallett attempts an answer by linking charity and reason through analytical philosophy.[19] He focuses on the criteria by which a Christian ethic based in charity can be judged. He posits a system of "Christian Moral Reasoning" that purports to reconcile the traditional allegiance to reason and objective norms with the concrete particulars involved in actual moral decisions. He proposes to avoid the absolutization of precepts he finds in traditional Christian ethics, on the one hand, and the abandonment of objective norms in the agapeistic situation ethics of Joseph Fletcher, on the other.

Hallett, thus, argues for a "third position" between the extremes of perceptive and antiperceptive ethics. This he calls value ethics, which makes use of the insights of analytical philosophy and judges the Christian nature of an act or decision by a balance of Christian values over disvalues. Hallett's concept of Christian value maximization is provocative and deserves further examination. His proposal is, however, largely procedural. It bypasses the substantive metaethical issues. He tries to give due preeminence to charity, even while denying the value of a specific hierarchy of values that would give the first place to charity. Earlier, William Spurrier developed a laudable comparative and compelling attempt at integration of Catholic natural-law theory and Protestant situation ethics. It is a synthesis of the objective and subjective demands of charity.[20]

An even more ambitious attempt to redefine Christian ethics comes from the "Murray Group"—theologians thinking, in the spirit of John Courtney Murray, from a "North American" viewpoint. They examine Catholic theology "through the eyes of American philosophy,"[21] by which they mean the philosophies of James, Dewey, Whitehead, Pierce, Royce, and especially Jonathan Edwards. From these sources they claim to derive a theology that not only is rational and objective but also takes into account the experiential, affective, aesthetic, and pragmatic dimensions of the moral life. They hope thus to balance the excessive rationalism they perceive in traditional Catholic moral philosophy by drawing on experience, feeling, and imagination.

This perspective is well represented by William Spohn,[22] who expands on the place of discernment and *metanoia* in making concrete ethical decisions by what he calls the reasoning heart. The reasoning heart does not contravene reasoning and moral principles in ethics. Rather, it operates within them but draws also on imagination and experience to illuminate individual moral decisions. "Discernment" says Spohn, "remains a personal search for the action of God in one's own history and in the events of the world. Although its conclusions are not morally generalizable, as judgments of rationality are, the reasoning heart of the Christian finds normative guidance in the symbols and story of revelation."[23] On this view, what distinguishes Christian ethics is that it is motivated, in the moment of moral choice, by a specific set of affections—those that most closely correspond to the character, affections, and goodness of Christ. Christian ethics differs from purely philosophical ethics because it can draw on these affections, which, without conversion, are closed to non-Christians.

This is not the place to enter into a detailed critique of this interesting mode of theologizing. Spohn recognizes the dangers of intuitionism and situationism in his approach. Just precisely how the balance is struck between moral sentiment and moral reason in this form of theology is not clear from Spohn's presentation or from the other essays in the anthology in which his appears. Like Hallett, Spohn is seeking a middle position between the extremes of fideism and rationalism. As with all middle positions, finding the precise point of balance is the crucial challenge.

Another linkage between philosophy and Christian belief is Norman Pittenger's application of Whitehead's process philosophy to the understanding of religious affirmation.[24] Pittenger examines the origins of Christian faith in humans as a Whiteheadean "event" and studies how, in Whitehead's terms, it apprehends the reality of Jesus and the way that reality opens "a window into God." Here, as with any interpretation of Christian belief in terms of a specific philosophical system, the links with more traditional ways of philosophizing need critical examination. With Whitehead or any of the other "North American" philosophical approaches, there is always a danger of eroding the still viable truths of a more traditional Catholic moral philosophy.

Pertinent to many of the attempts to balance affect and intellect in moral decisions are the current discussions on the relationships between moral cognition and moral motivation. Here the question is this: Does a recognition of the right and good impel to doing the right and good? Are these totally separable operations, and if they are not separable, how are they in fact linked?

Such questions are relevant to the nature of Christian ethics and to the various meanings of discernment as it is found in St. Ignatius, Karl Rahner, or the Murray Group. Some theorists suggest that moral motivation is a function of one's sense of self, rather than a function of one's conceptualization skills on the one hand or a matter of anticipations of external "bribes" and rewards on the other.[25] Conversion to the Christian faith creates St. Paul's "new man," one whose sense of self is shaped by the Christian virtues. Is this the way being a Christian makes a difference in ethics? Is it this transformation of the self that links cognition and motivation? Is this the locus for the "illumination" spoken of in the more classical moral theologians and the "discernment" preferred by their contemporary counterparts?

Each of these approaches attempts to reinterpret, in contemporary terms, the more traditional viewpoints on the relationships of philosophical and theological ethics as found in St. Augustine and St. Thomas. They are interesting in their own right, and they force us to seek a deeper understanding of the Catholic moral tradition. Thomas Gilbey reminds us that St. Thomas "jogs us to remember that philosophical ethics is contained within *sacra doctrina*, that the discourse is drawing from sources beyond the reach of reason alone, and that from within reason there is a reaching out to a good beyond reasonable statement, the ultimate good, transcendent yet not abstract, the burden of all yearning which is God himself, the end beyond measure of all morality."[26] St. Thomas' extended treatment of the human psychology of habit and passion gives a personalist cast to his ethics that should be reassuring to contemporary thinkers who fear the rigidity and absolutization of an exclusively prescriptive moral system. As Jan Walgrave points out, St. Thomas was "in his own way a personalist . . . because he combined a radical methodical intellectualism with a personalistic anti-rationalism, showing the radical insufficiency of ratiocination in determining the principles and in deciding the practical issues of moral life."[27]

In another recent series of studies, Servais Pinckaers shows how central to Thomistic ethics was the doctrine of charitable love as revealed in the Beatitudes.[28] Pinckaers traces the evolution and maturation of the idea of the good and its link with ethics, from the *finis bonorum* of Cicero, through Augustine's dictum that the Sermon on the Mount provided the "perfect pattern of the Christian life," to St. Thomas' own placement of the Beatitudes at the summit of Christian morality. The sure guide to happiness sought by the pagans as well as

Christians is the Beatitudes. Pinckaers sees in Thomas' interpretation the possibility of once more reconciling morality and the desire for happiness, which he sees divorced in contemporary ethics.

Pinckaers also takes the view that duties and obligations are secondary in the morality of St. Thomas. They are the "crutches" of the virtues, placed at their service: "La Morale de St. Thomas est donc une morale du bonheur et des vertus, groupant celles-ci autour de la foi, de la charité et des vertus cardinales. Ainsi s'explique le peu de place accordé dans la Somme à l'obligation morale."[29]

He goes on to show how during the Reformation and Counter Reformation, both Protestantism and Catholicism divorced morality and faith, the one in the direction of rejecting reason, the other in exalting the natural law. Both are misguided, says Pinckaers. If we wish to understand Thomistic ethics, we must restore the primary place to faith. The essential fact is the internal disposition to charitable action formed by faith and helped by the Holy Spirit. This, he holds, gives freedom, not arbitrariness, to Christian ethics.

In his reflection on the methodology of St. Thomas, Thomas O'Brien distinguishes St. Thomas' vision of beatitude from Aristotle's. For Aquinas beatitude is the result of union with God, not of virtuous activity as in Aristotle. The moral quality of human acts is, thus, measured by the degree to which they advance charity as the prime moral principle. Beatitude is a form of friendship and, therefore, of mutual love between God and man—a relationship that comes only through grace. "It is not, then, a question of seeing a natural moral structure, then filling it in by identifying the ultimate end as God; the vision of grace and charity is first; the moral structure is chosen to express something of its intelligibility."[30]

St. Thomas, thus, reverses the usual order of a naturalistic ethic, in which practice of the virtues can move man to his proper end of happiness. Instead, for Aquinas the only way to the fullness of beatitude is through grace and charity. Such fulfillment is for man "above the condition of his nature but not in disregard or negation of his nature."[31]

One of the more promising recent reexaminations of the philosophical foundations for Christian ethics is the interesting amalgam of Thomistic realism, Christian existentialism, and phenomenological methodology that goes under the heading of "Lublinism."[32] Here Christian ethics is grounded in the personalism of an ambitious philosophical anthropology. One of its most prominent exemplars is Karol

Wojtyla, now John Paul II, whose personalist ethics centers on the lived experience and participation in love of the acting person.[33] On that view, the traditional values of Catholic morality are preserved and enriched by some of the creative ideas in contemporary European philosophy.[34] This is in distinct contrast to both the analytical thrust of Anglo-American ethics and the legalistic bias of some Catholic moral theology in the past.

CONCLUSION

These recent attempts to bridge the gap between ethics as an enterprise of reason and ethics as fulfillment of the law of love are valuable extrapolations of the traditional Catholic perspective. They offer fresh insights into the links between philosophical and theological ethics, between contemporary and traditional ways of doing ethics, and between faith and reason, intellect and will, virtue and duties, agape and moral principles. We are far, however, from bridging all these gaps. An impressive new synthesis by Pinckaers of the old and new sources of Christian morality moves in this direction however.[35]

In all of this, it is important to avoid an overly eager acceptance of the new or an overly rigid adulation of the past. Intuitionism, situationism, psychologism, and biologism are easy traps to fall into. Yet the divisions between prescriptive and nonprescriptive ethics may not be as wide as their respective protagonists may feel. Those who favor existential and experiential modes of ethical thinking need a deeper and updated reacquaintance with Thomistic ethics. Those who favor the more traditional modes need to acquaint themselves with the richness of possible connections between Thomas' thought and contemporary philosophy and psychology.

The great strength of the thought of St. Augustine and St. Thomas lay in their capacity to engage in creative dialogue with the dominant cultural ideas of their times. Their intellects, illuminated by faith, were able to apprehend what was congruent with the law of charity and to discard what was not. If we can still philosophize and theologize in the spirit of Augustine and Thomas, it seems possible that a truly comprehensive Catholic medical moral philosophy will emerge. Such a philosophy would tell us more about the kinds of persons we ought to be than the rules we ought to follow. In medical morals it would call for Catholic health professionals who possess an intellectual grasp of moral principles as well as a capacity to apply them in the spirit of charity. In this way they might fulfill the law of love, which Guardini says "*is* the New Testament"[36] and without which Christian ethics is impossible.

NOTES

1. Joseph Fletcher, *Situation Ethics: The New Morality* (Philadelphia: Westminster Press, 1966).

2. Joseph Cardinal Ratzinger, "Magisterium of the Church, Faith, Morality," in *Readings in Moral Theology II: The Distinctiveness of Christian Ethics*, ed. Charles Curran and Richard McCormick (New York: Paulist Press, 1980), pp. 174–189.

3. John Ladd, "Internal Morality of Medicine: An Essential Dimension of the Patient-Physician Relationship," in *The Clinical Encounter*, ed. Earl Shelp (Dordrecht, Netherlands/Boston: D. Reidel, 1983), pp. 209–232.

4. John Paul II, *Encyclical Letter: Veritatis Splendor* (Washington: U.S. Catholic Conference, 1994).

5. Albert R. Jonsen and Stephen Toulmin, *The Abuse of Casuistry: A History of Moral Reasoning* (Berkeley: University of California Press, 1988).

6. Kevin D. O'Rourke and Philip Boyle, *Medical Ethics: Sources of Catholic Teachings*, 2d ed. (Washington: Georgetown University Press, 1993); Benedict M. Ashley and Kevin D. O'Rourke, *Health Care Ethics: A Theological Analysis*, 3d ed. (St. Louis: Catholic Health Association of the United States, 1989); Congregation for the Doctrine of the Faith, *Instruction on Respect for Human Life in Its Origin and on the Dignity of Procreation* (Washington: U.S. Catholic Conference, 1987); Orville Griese, *Catholic Identity in Health Care, Principles and Practice* (Braintree, Mass.: Pope John XXIII Center, 1987).

7. Alasdair MacIntyre, *Three Rival Versions of Moral Theory* (Notre Dame: University of Notre Dame Press, 1990), pp. 139–141; Edmund D. Pellegrino and David C. Thomasma, *The Virtues in Medical Practice* (New York: Oxford University Press, 1993).

8. Joseph Fuchs, "'Catholic' Medical Moral Theology?" in *Catholic Perspectives on Medical Morals*, ed. Edmund D. Pellegrino, John P. Langan, and John C. Harvey (Dordrecht, Netherlands/Boston: D. Reidel, 1989), pp. 83–92.

9. John Langan, "Moral Disagreements in Catholicism: A Commentary on Wallace, Schueller, and Thomasma," in *Catholic Perspectives*, ed. Pellegrino, Langan, and Harvey, pp. 79–80.

10. Robert Sokolowski, "The Art and Science of Medicine," in *Catholic Perspectives on Medical Morals*, ed. Pellegrino, Langan, and Harvey, pp. 263–276.

11. Edmund D. Pellegrino and David C. Thomasma, *A Philosophical Basis of Medical Practice* (New York: Oxford University Press, 1981).

12. Marcia Baron, "Kantian Ethics and Supererogation," *Journal of Philosophy* 84, no. 5 (1987): 237–262.

13. Lisa S. Cahill, "'Theological' Medical Morality: A Response to Joseph Fuchs," in *Catholic Perspectives*, ed. Pellegrino, Langan, and Harvey, pp. 93–102.

14. Philippa Foot, *Virtues and Vices* (Oxford: Basil Blackwell, 1978), pp. 12–14.

15. Romano Guardini, *The Lord* (Chicago: Regnery Press, 1954), p. 79.

16. Thomas Merton, *Love and Living* (New York: Harcourt Brace Jovanovich, 1985), p. 127.

17. William Frankena, *Ethics*, 2d ed. (Engelwood Cliffs, N.J.: Prentice-Hall, 1973), p. 58.

18. Frankena, *Ethics*, p. 57.

19. Garth L. Hallett, *Christian Moral Reasoning* (Notre Dame: University of Notre Dame Press, 1983).

20. William A. Spurrier, *Natural Law and the Ethics of Love* (Philadelphia: Westminster Press, 1974).

21. Frank M. Oppenheim, ed., *The Reasoning Heart* (Washington: Georgetown University Press, 1986).

22. William Spohn, "The Reasoning Heart: An American Approach to Christian Discernment," in *Reasoning Heart*, ed. Oppenheim, pp. 51-76.

23. Spohn, "Reasoning Heart," p. 56.

24. Norman Pittenger, *Catholic Faith in a Process Perspective* (Maryknoll, N.Y.: Orbis, 1981).

25. Thomas E. Wren, "Metaethical Internalism: Can Moral Beliefs Motivate?" *Proceedings of the American Catholic Philosophical Association* 59 (1985): 58–80.

26. Thomas Gilbey, "Appendix 6: Philosophical and Theological Morals," in St. Thomas Aquinas, *Summa Theologiae* [Vol. 18], ed. and trans. Thomas Gilbey (New York: Blackfriars, 1966), p. 147.

27. Jan H. Walgrave, "The Personal Aspects of St. Thomas' Ethics," in *Studi Tomistici*, ed. Leo J. Elders and Klaus Hedwig (Vatican City: Pontificia Academica, 1984), p. 214.

28. Servais Pinckaers, "Autonomie et hétéronomie en morale selon S. Thomas d'Aquin," in *Autonomie: Dimensions Éthiques de la liberté: Études d'éthique chrétienne* (Paris: Éditions du Cerf, 1983); "Le Commentaire du sermon sur la montagne par S. Augustin et la morale de S. Thomas d'Aquin," in *La teologia morale nella stroia e nella problematica Attaule miscellananea*, ed. Lawrence B. Gillon (Milan: Massimo, 1982), pp. 105–125; "La Béatitude dans l'éthique de S. Thomas," in *Studi Tomistici*, ed. Elders and Hedwig, pp. 80–94; and *Les Sources de la morale chrétienne: Sa methode, son contenu, son histoire*, 2d ed. (Fribourg, Switzerland: Éditions Universitaires, 1990).

29. Pinckaers, "Autonomie," p. 109.

30. Thomas C. O'Brien, "The *Reditus ad Deum:* A Reflection on the Methodology of St. Thomas," in St. Thomas Aquinas, *Summa Theologiae* [Vol. 27], ed. and trans. T. C. O'Brien (New York: Blackfriars, 1974), p. 114.

31. O'Brien, *"Reditus ad Deum,"* p. 97.

32. Karol Wojtyla, *The Acting Person*, [*Analecta Husserliana* X], trans. Andrezej Potocki (Dordrecht, Netherlands: D. Reidel, 1979); Mieczyslaw A. Krapiec, *I-Man: An Outline of Philosophical Anthropology* (New Britain, Conn.: Mariel, 1983); Ronald D. Lawler, "Personalist Ethics," *Proceedings of the American Catholic Philosophical Association* 60 (1986): 148–155.

33. Wojtyla, *The Acting Person;* Kenneth L. Schmitz, *At the Center for the Human Drama: The Philosophical Anthropology of Karol Wojtyla/Pope John Paul II* (Washington: Catholic University of America, 1993).

34. Emmanuel Levinas, *Otherwise than Being; or, Beyond Essence,* trans. Alphonso Lingis (Boston: Kluwer, 1981); Max Scheler, *Man's Place in Nature,* trans. Hans Meyerhoff (New York: Noonday Press, 1961); Martin Buber, *I and Thou,* trans. Ronald Gregor Smith (New York: Scribners, 1986).

35. Pinckaers, *Les Sources de la morale chrétienne;* Servais Pinckaers, *Universalité et permanence des lois morales* (Fribourg, Switzerland: Éditions Universitaires, 1986).

36. Guardini, *The Lord,* p. 79.

3

The Virtue of Faith

Sacred to the Memory of Doctor Zabdiel Boston, esq., Physician and Fellow of the Royal Society. Through a life of extreme beneficence he was always faithful to his word, just in his dealings, affable in his manners; & after a long sickness in which he was exemplary for his patience and resignation to his Maker he quitted this Mortal Life in a just expectation of happy Immortality on the first day of March A.D. 1766 Aetatis 87.

–A Tombstone in Brookline, Massachusetts[1]

"Faith is man's response to God Who reveals Himself to man at the same time bringing man a superabundant light as he searches for the ultimate meaning of his life."[2] This is the way the new *Catechism* begins and the way it inaugurates its compendium of the whole way of life to which Catholic Christians—indeed, all men and women—are called. Faith is the inaugural virtue. It opens the way to the truth and points to the path that leads to salvation.

Once the path is shown to us by faith, then hope helps us to persevere on the way, and charity binds us so firmly to that way that we are not willing to lose it for any other good or in order to avoid any harm. Thus, faith is the first of the supernatural virtues, the helmsman that keeps us from pursuing the wrong byways or attaching ourselves to the wrong goods or even to evils. Faith is our spiritual compass.

Faith is also a complex virtue. Sometimes we make our act of faith in the midst of despair to bridge the gap between what we experience and the mystery of what that experience means in the divine order. Sometimes faith offers the answer; sometimes, only more mystery. Sometimes it comforts; sometimes it pains. Sometimes it is distorted by bigotry, scrupulosity, or presumption. Faith is a gift of God that both circumscribes and, at the same time, enhances our human capacities. As Jesus said, "If you have faith, you can move mountains."

The desire to believe is a natural human propensity. We could not trust one another without it. We could not talk with one another without the expectation that we will be believed or that the other person has the capacity to understand us. Every time we fly, cross a bridge, or submit to general anesthesia, we exhibit our faith in human capabilities. But the mystery of faith as it is manifest in the supernatural virtue is infinitely more profound. It is nothing less than a response to a call to perfection, to happiness we ourselves cannot attain without God's grace, to a partnership with God in all our endeavors. Jews and Christians believe they live in a covenantal partnership with God, in a dialogue with the Creator in which humans cocreate their institutions and civilizations with God's help.

One reason the virtue of faith is so complex is that it touches both the mind and the will of the believer, requiring a change in life and a difference in conduct. In Hebrews 11:1 the virtue of faith is defined as "the substance of things to be hoped for, the evidence of things unseen." St. Thomas defends the conjunction of the will and intellect embodied in this definition: "The act of faith is belief, an act of mind fixed on one alternative by reason of the will's command. This implies that the act of faith has a reference both to the will's object, i.e., the good or end, and to the mind's object, i.e., the true. And because faith is a theological virtue, having the one reality as its object and its end, it follows necessarily that the object of faith and its end stand in a mutual relationship."[3]

Moreover, Judeo-Christian faith focuses on the living God who is trusted, who is the first unseen and mysterious truth and the object of hope. Thus, the primary focus of faith is on the personhood of God. A person of faith is related not only to all around him or her but also to the creating and redeeming God. Faith calls forth the love of others, hope for the eventual good, prudence about applying fundamental moral principles to new situations, compassion for the sick and the vulnerable, generosity of time and effort for others, and a host of other virtues.

Faith acknowledges the sovereignty of God over the universe and our lives. It moves us to trust in his exercise of that sovereignty even when we cannot comprehend its operation in the world and in our lives. If we have faith, we surrender our whole being to God's dominion. We do not, and cannot, have true faith and still wrest that dominion from God by trying to control every facet of our own lives or forcing our faith on others. Faith is a free gift of God. Those who do not have it, for reasons we cannot discern, have not been granted it by God. We usurp God's sovereignty when we force our faith on another by tyranny, crusade, or coerced conversion. When people of faith in the past have justified their faith this way, they were really showing that they themselves did not have faith but an ideological simulacrum of faith.

Faith also reveals to us a new world in which we become new men and women. Faith is God's gift nurtured by fidelity to the good news of the Gospel. It is by faith that our intellects are assured that what God asks of us is the wish of a good, loving, and forgiving Creator, a Father whose intent our limited minds can never fathom completely. Faith enables us to perdure, even when God appears to be punishing us, or those we love, and seems to be unjust and asking more of us than we can bear.

This is preeminently the case when illness, disability, and death afflict us and our loved ones. Illness is one of the few remaining things over which humans do not have full dominion. The vaunted powers of medicine notwithstanding, we know we will all ultimately sicken and die, sometimes in unpleasant and even horrible ways. The challenge of human suffering is the ultimate challenge to faith in a good and all-powerful God for both the patient and the physician. The temptation to question, doubt, and despair is ever present. Paradoxically, while misfortune challenges faith, it is only faith that can give hope and meaning to human suffering and dying. As C. S. Lewis says, an act of faith is a transforming act: "It is to change from being confident about our own efforts to the state in which we despair of doing anything for ourselves and leave it to God."[4]

The believer also realizes that in faith he acknowledges his dependence on God even while he can never penetrate the mystery of the challenge to our hope and love in the events of our daily lives. The physician, despite the challenge of this mystery to his scientific training, nonetheless accepts the mystery. He practices his healing art, but knows that the grasp of the full meaning of illness and healing will not be his. Faith reveals itself therefore in humility but not in pusillanimity. We continue to strive to heal, to relieve suffering, to bring our knowledge to bear on the illness and the patient. But we know also that God works within us and within his creation and that we do not heal by our own power alone.[5]

The Christian physician, then, is not ashamed to pray, to ask God to show how to heal in this case, how to use medical knowledge to heal, how to make the patient whole again in body, mind, and spirit. The physician does not fear to pray with the patient, to call upon the patient's spiritual resources, or to ask the chaplain's assistance. The committed Christian, doctor or not, gives witness to faith through humility before the unfathomable uniqueness of the mystery in the predicament of a patient's illness.

Ultimately, it is by the virtue of faith, as much as doctrines or dogmas, important as these may be, that the physician "puts on the new man." Acceptance of the mystery is the first step to penetrating the mystery. Out of this acceptance, the anointing of the sick, and the powerful sacrament of hope grows the capacity to hope for the good when all seems evil and to love God and man and self in God. It is in this capacity to love and hope when all seems lost that true faith consists.

THE CHRISTIAN PHYSICIAN—HISTORICAL ORIGINS

From its beginnings, medicine has been inextricably entwined with religion, with belief in some transcendent order with which humans must engage, either in denial or affirmation. In short, with some faith commitment. This faith was first placed in the pagan deities, then in the God of the monotheistic religions of Christianity, Judaism, and Islam. In the past, this faith was challenged by a multiplicity of heresies and the resurgent pull to paganism. In the modern era this faith was eroded for many people by the post-Enlightenment move to rationalism, agnosticism, and atheism. But a persistent religious perspective on healing has survived despite these erosive tendencies.

Medicine itself had its origins in primitive religious beliefs, in the presumption that illness was in some way the result of inimical forces—the intrusion into the body of some foreign object or hostile spirit, the robbing of one's soul, or punishment for violation of sacred taboos.[6] These were, and remain, the basis for the notions of pathogenesis and the therapeutics of the medicine man, shaman, and folk healer. They persist in the unconscious as archaic remnants that surface in times of very great stress. The contribution of the ancient Greeks was to make medicine both a rational and an ethical enterprise.

The first commitment was to make medicine a rational activity. This meant it had to be distanced from its magico-religious origins; it had to seek its causes in natural phenomena and thus make healing itself a natural enterprise.[7] Early physicians spoke of the *vis medicatrix naturae*, the healing force of nature. Whereas early religious medicine had looked to spirits and magic to heal, the Hippocratic physician turned to restoration of the body's own healing powers.

But interestingly, even as Greek medicine declared itself free from religion and identified itself as a craft or *teknē*,[8] it still called upon the gods for its healing powers (the Hippocratic oath).[9] Hippocratic physicians were followers of Aesculapius. They healed in temples such as those at Cos and Epidaurus and committed themselves to a virtuous way of life. They required the same of aspirants to the profession, who were expected to make a commitment to medicine as a special calling dedicated to the interests of the sick.

This ethical commitment to the welfare of the sick person was the second great contribution of Hippocratic medicine. It gave medicine a perduring ethical framework. It united physicians into a moral community with shared ethical ideals and a way of life dedicated to beneficence and nonmaleficence, avoidance of abortion and euthanasia, protection of confidentiality, and a promise not to take sexual advantage of the vulnerability of patients and families.

This ethical tradition was amplified in later centuries by the Stoic physicians, particularly those of the Middle and Later Stoa. Stoicism contributed the ethics of obligations and duties. It emphasized the shared humanity of all peoples and, for the first time, made healing a profession, one based in compassion and mercy for the sick. Some of the later Stoic writers expressed sentiments of love for the patient, identification with his or her suffering, and disdain for financial gain that are very close to the sentiments that should motivate the Christian physician.[10]

Despite these noble aspirations and counsels of pagan medicine, the most profound transformation in what it meant to be a healer came when Christianity became an influence on the culture of the ancients. Henry Sigerist, the distinguished social historian of medicine, put it well: "It remained to Christianity to introduce the most revolutionary change in the attitude of society toward the sick. Christianity came into the world as the religion of healing, as the joyful Gospel of the Redeemer and the Redemption."[11] Sigerist goes on to describe how Christianity removed the stigma of punishment from illness and gave the sick a preferential position they had never enjoyed in the pagan world. The result was a transformation of the pagan Hippocratic ethic by the spirit of charity, the ordering virtue of the Christian physician.

The roots of the change effected in care of the sick by Christians were firmly planted in the Hebrew Bible and the teachings of Jesus. In the former, the scriptural texts taught that healing is from God (Exodus 15:26, Job 5:18, Hosea 7:1, Deuteronomy 7:15, and Jeremiah 17:14). Sirach 38:1–15 is particularly apposite. Sirach tells us that we must honor the physician because we have need of him, but we must also recognize that his healing power comes from God. Even the medicines the doctor uses were placed in the earth by God. Even with these medicines, the author of the Book of Sirach advises us not to ignore prayer, sacrifice, and spiritual cleansing.

These obligations to heal and to care for the sick in the Jewish Bible were expanded in a new direction by the teachings of the Gospel. The unprecedented facts of the Incarnation, Atonement, and Resurrection gave new meanings to illness, suffering, and healing. Jesus' life was devoted to teaching the way of salvation, but also to healing. There are thirty-five instances of healing in the Gospels, wherein Jesus shows his and the Father's solicitude for suffering. Jesus himself suffered and died according to the will of the Father, surrendering his spirit to that will in the last moment of his life. He was, indeed, the "wounded healer" of whom Isaiah spoke.[12]

Jesus lived his whole life in fulfillment of the words of Leviticus 19:18: "You shall love your neighbor as yourself." In the way Jesus fulfilled these words, we are shown the meaning of the virtue of Christian charity, one that goes beyond pagan notions of *philia, humanitas,* or *misericordia.*[13]

On this view, being sick was no longer a disgrace, a public sign of individual sin, as Job's friends had so belligerently insisted. Rather, illness came to be accepted as the result of Original Sin shared by the whole of humanity (John 9:2–3, 11:4). To suffer was to follow in the way of the Master.[14] The sick person was not to be rejected but was owed a special level of solicitude. The Christian was to see Christ in every suffering man and woman (Romans 12:15; 2 Corinthians 1, 2, 7, 10).[15]

In subsequent centuries, the revolutionary message of the Gospels and Epistles was greeted with varying degrees of acceptance.[16] Some of the early Christians were particularly concerned about how the use of physicians could be reconciled with faith in the healing powers of prayer, anointing, and laying of hands, or even whether Christian physicians could swear the Hippocratic oath. These tensions were more or less resolved by the third century A.D. By then, the Christian community, the religious communities, and the institutional church had accepted and encouraged the care of the sick as a necessary and admirable apostolate. Out of that apostolate grew the religious foundation of hospitals, hospices, and homes for the care of the sick, the poor, the aged, and the orphaned with which we associate the ideal of Christian charity and the corporal works of mercy.

Today the idea of the Christian physician is an amalgam of the ethical commitments to the sick by the Hippocratic physicians, the divine revelations of Jewish and Christian Scripture, the tradition of healing as an apostolate of all Christians, and a coterminous commitment to scientific competence. For the Christian, this whole amalgam is transmuted by faith into a way of serving God and one's fellows. The tension that some see in this alliance of diverse elements of disparate provenance is made constructive rather than destructive by the Christian's belief in the unity of all creation under the parenthood of God.

CHALLENGES TO THE HIPPOCRATIC-CHRISTIAN SYNTHESIS

In the last quarter century, this tradition has come under serious challenge by seven opposing traditions, which have incubated through the centuries but have never been as influential as they are today.[17] These are the traditions of secular humanism, scientism and positivism, technological medicine, entrepreneurism, philosophical relativism, moral atomism, and pragmatism. Each poses a serious threat to the traditional ideal of the Christian physician in both its components, the Hippocratic and the Christian.

Let us begin first with a brief recitation of the sociocultural and philosophical origins of the threats to the tradition.

A primary eroding force is the progressive loss of religious faith, for it destroys the central core of what it is to be a Christian physician. In denying the reality of God, of Jesus Christ, and of the Bible, the whole substructure of moral validation for the tradition is demolished. On this view, Christ and his teaching, however admirable, are merely stories among other stories. There is no way to give them special moral weight. Humans, therefore, are the source of morality. The idea, therefore, of any source of medical morality outside what is politically negotiable is simply rejected out of hand. Thus, the idea of a universal or objective order of medical ethics is meaningless. Dostoyevsky's Aloysha was right: when God is dead, everything is, indeed, possible.

The second source of erosion is the power of empirical science and the positivistic philosophy it nurtures. On this view, all talk of ethics or morals is about mere opinion unverifiable by factual demonstration. Instead of looking to religion or even philosophy for moral directives, some would look to biology. Ethics is merely a phenomenon of population biology, of neurobiology—of an evolutionary device that is valuable simply because it permits survival of the gene pool. Ethics should be literally "bio-ethics"—that is to say, biological ethics —observable, quantifiable, even demonstrable as part of biological science and in accord with Darwinian evolutionary theory.[18] Sometimes this view is conflated with a cousin, sociobiology.

Positivism leads to technicism—the conviction that all of life can ultimately be regulated and controlled by technological prowess. The age of the computer encourages many to think that the whole of medicine is reducible to algorithms. In this third view, the desirable future is one in which the physician is wholly or partially replaced. The patient no longer need worry about the doctor's character, the vagaries of his or her personality, or the misuse of the power that knowledge confers. This is, indeed, the nirvana of those who would absolutize autonomy. In this new world, there is no place, no need indeed, for the Hippocratic or Christian physician who would dare to help a patient and act in the interest of that patient.

A fourth erosive force is the rise of entrepreneurism as a self-justifying enterprise reducing all human activity to self-interest with the same irresistibility the Freudians ascribe so confidently to the libido. Economics, instead of being a means to an end—literally, "housekeeping"—becomes the determinant of all social values, a definer of the kind of society and professions we should have. When economics and entrepreneurism drive the professions, they admit only self-interest and the working of the marketplace as the motives for professional activity. In a free-market economy, effacement of self-interest, or any conduct shaped primarily by the idea of altruism or virtue, is simply inconsistent with survival. Health care is just another commodity provided by the physician, who is a worker in the health care "industry." The quality, quantity, price, availability, accessibility, and kind of health care are simply resultants of the operation of the "invisible hand" of the marketplace. Conflict of interest results.

A fifth factor eroding the tradition of the Christian physician is philosophical relativism and the deconstruction of the whole of philosophy that has been taking place gradually for several centuries. Metaphysics was eradicated a long time ago when philosophers gave up the search for the really real. Epistemology followed when we gave up any hope of knowing something about the external world beyond the content of our own minds. Now ethics has abandoned the search for moral truth, satisfying itself with an analysis of the way we talk about morality, or simply describing the different ways we justify moral beliefs, or simply tallying up the consensus among ethicists—at least those deemed creditable by the opinion makers. Philosophy has become merely a conversation in which we swap vaguely remembered stories of disparate provenance, all equally believable no matter how outrageous. Of course, the one story ignored is the story of God and his conversation through time with his people—a conversation with some definite instructions about right conduct that are not susceptible to change by a new consensus of the cognoscenti.

Whenever philosophy is eroded, theology invariably goes with it. Philosophy cannot avoid abutting on the question of God. The pagan philosophers—Plato, Aristotle, the Stoics — could not avoid natural theology. Today even nonbelievers—and some believers—are yielding to New Age pressures, to that Neo-Gnostic, secular religion whose high priests tell us not only what is politically but what is philosophically correct.

A sixth factor is the growing displacement of the communitarian ethic by the ethic of moral atomism, privatism, and untrammeled individualism.[19] This is a natural outgrowth of the doctrine of negative rights contained in the philosophy of John Locke in his *Second Treatise Concerning Government*. For Locke, and for Hobbes as well, society was created by a contract freely entered into by individuals for the sake of mutual protection against each other. The idea that society was natural and necessary for human fulfillment, as Aristotle argued, was discarded as unrealistic. The absolutization of autonomy, the libertarian cast of politics and ethics, and the balkanization of private morals as irrelevant to the good of society are outgrowths of the triumph of individualism.

The seventh factor, and the last we mention, is the very subtle strain of pragmatism that infects even the physician who is a Christian and, by that fact, leads to a compromise of faith in the name of exigency. By this we mean the quiet acquiescence in the separation of private beliefs from professional ethics—as if the gospel could be sealed in the home and church and kept out of the agora. Here we point only to the complacent Christian who does not want to stand out, who is prosperous and successful, who mistakes moral flaccidity for tolerance, whose practice has no poor people, whose income is unconscionable, whose lifestyle is indistinguishable from those of his or her secular counterparts, who insists that he or she could not survive unless he or she, too, "protects" self-interest and becomes a part of the health or medical-industrial complex.

These are some of the powerful forces—and there are others at work today—disassembling the Hippocratic-Christian tradition and substituting the ideals of the physician as secular humanist, technician, entrepreneur, manager of health care, or autonomous "provider" dealing with consumers and clients, who are not patients any longer but parties to a contract rather than a covenant.[20]

As a result, the Hippocratic ethic has been cleansed of what many think are its moral pretensions. Medicine is no longer a moral community; beneficence has been replaced by autonomy as the first principle of ethics; abortion is, and euthanasia and assisted suicide will soon be, prescriptions rather than proscriptions; for some, sexual intercourse with patients may be part of the therapeutic regimen; and the idea of a "pure" or virtuous life as the life of the good physician is a matter of increasing ridicule.

With the Hippocratic component dismantled, the Christian component is even more easily destroyed. Religion is reduced to a series of comforting stories; Christ is reduced to an admirable but impractical model; healing, to a technical exercise; and prayer, to superstition. If one insists on being religious, for heaven's sake, do not bring it into professional life, and certainly not into public life! Often, to be identified as a Christian physician is to be disenfranchised, to be excluded from the debate as "unreasonable," and to be discounted as intellectually suspect or effete. Physicians who espouse Christianity today must live in a world in which the tradition of a Christian physician is diminished, ridiculed, and depreciated. Yet, paradoxically, perhaps there has never been a time when the difference that being a Christian makes to being a physician was more important. What difference does a faith commitment make in today's medical milieu? That is the question we address throughout the book.

FAITH'S INFLUENCE ON PRACTICE AND ETHICS

What difference does the virtue of faith make in the way a physician approaches the practice of medicine and in the way he or she interprets the moral obligations of a physician? No precise formula is sufficient to answer these questions. Indeed, the answers are convincingly manifest only in concrete clinical situations in which the Christian physician is called upon to be both a healer and a Christian healer.

Faith orients the healer to the way in which the practice of healing becomes charitable healing, i.e., an act of love performed in the manner of Christ's healing. Faith keeps before the healer his or her ultimate end and that of the patient. Faith restrains the hubris technology so easily engenders in today's physician or nurse. When hope flags, faith calls to mind that the purpose of human existence is union with God, not immortality or freedom from pain and suffering. Faith restores hope, even in the face of an incurable illness, not because cure of the illness is less a good but because faith promises more than cure. It invites belief in a good even higher than cure because God has promised that higher good to those who suffer.

The natural virtues of medicine that we have adumbrated in an earlier work—benevolence, fidelity to trust, compassion, intellectual honesty, self-effacement[21]—are all reshaped by the supernatural virtue of faith for both the believing physician and the believing patient.

To be sure, the Christian physician must exhibit these natural virtues of medicine as a healing art because these virtues are good in themselves. They are necessary dispositions to good healing. They are not erased by faith or replaced by the supernatural virtues. Rather, they receive added meaning because they are good in the order of nature created by God. Through faith all the virtues of the good physician are prefigured by the healing example of Christ himself.

As a result, benevolence extends beyond avoiding harm, or even simply doing good. It requires doing good at some sacrifice to oneself. Effacement of self-interest becomes an act of charity. Pro bono care of the poor and the elderly is not merely a legal or moral option. It is a way the Christian is expected to respond to the vulnerable and the neglected members of the human community. Compassion becomes a genuine sharing of the suffering of another. Intellectual honesty becomes a matter of the humility required of a created being before the mystery of illness and healing. Clinical prudence embraces clinical judgment but also the capacity to discern causes of pain and suffering not manifest in physiological responses, and the way best to alleviate those causes. Reform of the health care system must always be guided by the goal of improving the healing relationship with fellow creatures of God. Fidelity to trust becomes a sacred obligation to protect the well-being of the sick person.[22] Faith, in short, is a lantern that illuminates the way all the natural medical virtues should be lived by Christian physicians.

Faith is also the spiritual compass we need in the face of the moral and ethical dilemmas of modern medical practice. Faith entails a commitment to a source of morality beyond humankind, a source in Sacred Scripture, tradition, the teachings of the church and of its official magisterium. In a recent encyclical, *Veritatis Splendor*,[23] Pope John Paul II definitively set forth the fundamental presuppositions upon which a faith-directed response to ethical issues should be based. The purpose of this encyclical was "to set forth with regard to the problems being discussed, the principles of moral teaching based on Sacred Scripture, and the living apostolic tradition and at the same time to shed light on the presuppositions and consequences of the dissent which that teaching has met."[24]

Veritatis Splendor is too important and too prophetic a document for brief summarization here. Its implications for both the content and the method of conducting the enterprise of medical ethics are of the utmost significance to Catholic Christian physicians. In *Veritatis Splendor*, His Holiness reaffirms the centrality of faith in ethical deliberations and the place of the magisterium in the discernment of current "theological and cultural trends."[25]

These trends are particularly urgent and divisive even among Christians, particularly as they relate to the human-life issues of abortion, voluntary euthanasia, assisted suicide, and a variety of reproductive and genetic manipulations. The growth of subjectivism and relativism and the move to socially constructed ethics pose serious challenges to any form of Christian ethics. The response of John Paul II to these "tendencies" demonstrates their incompatibility with faith and revealed truth. It is the response of the overarching gospel imperative to the rich young man's question to the Lord: "What must I do to gain eternal life"?[26]

The precise implications of the encyclical for moral theology, ethics in general, and medical ethics in particular are outside the scope of this book. At this juncture in our inquiry into the supernatural virtues, it is necessary to understand the emphasis the encyclical places on fidelity to the foundations of the faith. These foundations are, as they have always been, in the Sacred Scriptures and church teaching. Faith in these foundations now, as always, illumines the difficult and often uncharted pathways of contemporary ethical discourses and decisions.

The Catholic Christian has the clear responsibility to become well informed in what faith teaches and to give witness to it in his or her own daily practice. Without the infused virtue of faith, this task is beyond the natural virtues of medicine.

NOTES

1. Thomas C. Mann and Janet Greene, *Over Their Dead Bodies: Yankee Epitaphs and History* (New York: Barnes and Noble, 1993), p. 12.

2. *Catechism of the Catholic Church* (New York: Paulist Press, 1994), p. 13.

3. St. Thomas Aquinas, *Summa Theologiae* [Vol. 13], trans. Thomas C. O'Brien (New York: Blackfriars, 1974), II-II, q. 4, a. 1, pp. 112–119.

4. Charles S. Lewis, *The Joyful Christian* (New York: Macmillan, 1977), p. 134.

5. Sirach, chap. 38, in *The New American Bible* (New York: Catholic Book Publishing, 1970), pp. 807–808.

6. Henry Sigerist, *A History of Medicine* [Vol. 1] (New York: Oxford University Press, 1951), pp. 125–191.

7. Hippocrates, *Ancient Medicine*, trans. W. H. S. Jones [Loeb Classical Library] (Cambridge: Harvard University Press, 1972), pp. 13–63.

8. Hippocrates, *Ancient Medicine*, pp. 13–63.

9. Hippocrates, *Ancient Medicine*, pp. 299–301.

10. Edmund D. Pellegrino and Alice A. Pellegrino, "Humanism and Ethics in Roman Medicine: Translation and Commentary on a Text of Scribonius Largus," *Literature and Medicine: Literature and Bioethics* 7 (1988): 22–38.

11. Henry E. Sigerist, *Civilization and Disease* (Ithaca, N.Y.: Cornell University Press, 1944), p. 69.

12. Isaiah, chaps. 42, 49, and 50, in *The New American Bible.*

13. See chapter 5 on the virtue of charity.

14. St. Gregory the Great, *Morals on the Book of Job* [Vol. 1] (Oxford: John Henry Parker, 1844).

15. Benedict M. Ashley and Kevin D. O'Rourke, *Ethics of Health Care* (St. Louis: Catholic Health Association of the United States, 1986).

16. Owsei Temkin, *Hippocrates in a World of Pagans and Christians* (Baltimore: Johns Hopkins University Press, 1991); Darrell Amundsen and Gary Ferngren, "The Early Christian Tradition," in *Caring and Curing*, ed. Ronald Numbers and Darrell Amundsen (New York: Macmillan, 1986), pp. 40–64.

17. Portions of this section appeared in C. S. Campbell and B. A. Lustig, eds., *Duties to Others* (Dordrecht, Netherlands/Boston: Kluwer, 1994).

18. Indeed, in its early days, it was so named by Van R. Potter in his *Bioethics: Bridge to the Future* (Engelwood Cliffs, N.J.: Prentice-Hall, 1971).

19. Erich H. Loewy, *Suffering and the Beneficent Community* (Buffalo: State University of New York Press, 1991).

20. David C. Thomasma, "Models of the Doctor-Patient Relationship and the Ethics Committee, Part I," *Cambridge Quarterly of Health Care Ethics* 1, no. 1 (1992): 11–31; and "Models of the Doctor-Patient Relationship and the Ethics Committee, Part II," *Cambridge Quarterly of Health Care Ethics* 3, no. 1 (1994): 10–26.

21. Edmund D. Pellegrino and David C. Thomasma, *For the Patient's Good: The Restoration of Beneficence in Health Care* (New York: Oxford University Press, 1988).

22. Edmund D. Pellegrino, "Trust and Distrust in Professional Ethics," in *Ethics, Trust, and the Professions: Philosophical and Cultural Aspects*, ed. Edmund D. Pellegrino, Robert M. Veatch, and John P. Langan (Washington: Georgetown University Press, 1991), pp. 69–89.

23. Pope John Paul II, *Papal Encyclical: Veritatis Splendor* (Washington: U.S. Catholic Conference, 1994).

24. Pope John Paul II, *Veritatis Splendor*, p. 11.

25. Pope John Paul II, *Veritatis Splendor*, p. 113.

26. Pope John Paul II, *Veritatis Splendor*, p. 113. The moral encounter, the question of the young man, the response offered by Jesus, and the tragic ending of this story all parallel the many daily choices facing professionals today.

4

Hope and Healing

> *Hope has for its object only what is good, and only what is future, and only what affects the person who entertains the hope.*
>
> — St. Augustine, *The Enchiridion.*[1]

Faith points the way, hope sustains us on that way. Every physician and nurse, indeed every observant person, knows that hope is essential to healing. When either the physician or the patient loses hope, the will to be healed is eroded. Illness then establishes its hegemony over the patient's mind and body. Despair, disability, depression, or death must then supervene. How hope is nurtured and how it is killed are thus central to understanding the predicament of illness and to shaping our efforts to help those caught in that predicament. This chapter will look at the phenomenon of hope—at what role it plays in healing, in what hope consists, in what ways it influences the responses to illness and recovery, and what ethical responsibilities the nurturing of hope imposes on those who offer to help the sick professionally or simply as friends or family members.

HOPE AS A NATURAL PHENOMENON

Humans cannot live without hope, without the conviction that some good they desire is possible of attainment, albeit with difficulty.[2] Hope was considered by the medieval philosophers as an emotion, a passion, that focuses on a *bonum arduum*, a good in the future that we desire but that is surrounded by obstacles.[3] We do not hope for things we are sure of getting. When we are certain we will overcome the intervening obstacles, hope is unnecessary. Hope is the belief, in the face of obstacles, that what we desire will be ours although we realize there is danger that our desire will not be fulfilled. Virgil suggests that this combination of hope and fear "permit[s] the fearful to have hope."[4] Thus, hope is a kind of courage about life. As Madeleine Vaillot puts it: "Hope is in essence a psychic commitment to life and growth, the ability to believe that one will feel better in the future, and the pervasive force which stimulates the system to actively seek new experiences and exposure to new forces in an attempt to achieve the highest level of behavioral functioning. Hope sustains the system through periods of disequilibrium."[5]

Hope is a mean between presumption and despair.[6] Presumption unwisely underestimates the impediments between us and the good we desire. Despair, on the other hand, is the abandonment of our conviction that the obstacles might or could ever be overcome. Despair in its severest form is a retreat from the desire and from the good that is the object of desire. Hope is a motivating force essential to any human endeavor. It goes beyond merely taking possession of what is readily at hand. Despair is loss of that motivation. To take up any task without the conviction that it is possible of attainment is to fail from the outset. But the more one possesses hope, the greater are the obstacles one can overcome.[7]

Hope is inextricably tied to love and faith. Whether the future good we desire is a person, thing, or place, we must first desire or love something. Without an object, hope is meaningless. Also, we must have faith, i.e., some projection of belief in possibilities beyond what is immediately obvious to logic or observation. We shall see later how hope as a spiritual virtue is also inextricable from the spiritual virtues of charity and faith, which characterize the religious perspective on the experience and ethics of healing.

Gabriel Marcel pointed out an interesting distinction between "I hope . . ." and, "I hope that . . ."[8] The latter is a statement people make frequently in everyday life. Here hope is expressed in relation to a specific concrete and definable desire. "I hope . . ." is a more general cosmic conviction about the possibility of hope in the human life or being in general. This is hope about the meaningfulness and purpose of human existence. This is the dimension of hope that existentialists like Camus or Sartre reject when they speak of the absurdity of the universe in which humanity is condemned to live without hope. Sisyphus is Camus' prototype of existential despair—humanity endlessly rolling a stone uphill only to have it roll down, again and again, ad infinitum.[9]

Illness (i.e., subjective perception of disease) and disease (i.e., the objective, medically apprehended signs of pathology) challenge both kinds of hope. Let us look at the concrete phenomenon of hope as it is present in the healing relationship.

BECOMING ILL OR DISABLED

What is the meaning of being ill? Most people regard themselves to be in a state of health. A state of health cannot be determined absolutely. Despite all the recent attempts to define health, no better functional definition of health has been given than by Galen, who defined health as that state "in which we neither suffer pain nor are hindered in the functions of daily life."[10] But this means that one can feel in a state of health and feel well, even while one may have disease. Indeed, many of us have undetected disease within us and yet are able to do the things we want to do with a minimum of discomfort and disability. Judging our own health and illness is considerably subjective. One person may have absolutely nothing wrong with him, may have been checked over for days in a medical center, and still feel and look sick. Another may have just learned that she has a treatment-responsive form of Hodgkin's disease, and be pleased that she did not have a more unrelenting form of cancer. The former is doing well, but feeling worse; the latter is doing worse, but feeling well. Still another may have just completed an extensive checkup without discovery of pathology and die suddenly two days later. This person is looking well, feeling well, and at the brink of death.

Thus, the ancients were correct in characterizing health as a state of balance. We become ill when something happens that shakes us out of that feeling of being in a healthy state and prompts us to seek help. That balance is upset by some symptom: a pain in the chest, the finding of a lump, a sore that does not heal, loss of appetite, morning nausea, dizziness on bending over. When these symptoms are perceived as a change in the function of our whole organism, they become sufficient to lead us to seek help. We become patients when we need help in bearing a problem, a pain, a concern, an anxiety. Actually, it makes no difference whether the problem is emotional or physical; when we seek professional help, we become patients. In becoming patients we enter a new existential state of dependency and vulnerability. In this state of vulnerability called illness, the body becomes the center of our concern because it is an impediment to, rather than a willing instrument for, the things we want to do. The self is reduced to an ego and a body.[11] The task of healing is a response to this dissolution.

As Eric Cassell cautions, a sick person is not merely "a well person with the knapsack of illness strapped to his back" but a newly constituted human entity in need. One of the main functions of healing this dissolution of the person into the ego and body, then, is to reconstitute the patient's integrity as a person, a self-governing entity, and this means enhancing the patient's autonomy.[12] But it also means providing hope that, in fact, the predicament of illness can be ameliorated or cured.

HOPE, ILLNESS, DISEASE

There are ways in which illness and disease may eventuate in good, but patients do not know this at the outset of the encounter with sickness. Even if they did, few would seek to be ill for this reason. For most people, illness is an evil—the absence of a good, namely, health. When we seek medical or health care, we desire restoration of a good we perceive we have lost. Health is the *bonum arduum*, the difficult-to-reach good, that is the object of the patient's hope. Sick persons appreciate that there may be many obstacles to fulfillment of their hopes. The disease may be chronic and ameliorable but not curable.[13] The probabilities of a good or a bad outcome cannot be known with certainty in advance. Many other obstacles are possible—cost, availability, accessibility, a physician's limited skills, the inherent fallibilities of medical techniques, the side effects and toxicity of medications, etc.

To be healed in the face of these uncertainties, we must be motivated by hope.[14] To set out on the sometimes perilous and uncertain journey of medical treatment, we must have hope that the good of health will be attained. Without hope few would embark on what may be an arduous, painful, and unsuccessful venture.[15] Hope is needed even after we set out. We need hope to sustain us in those dark moments when the goal is in doubt or the destination becomes less attractive than it was at the outset.[16] For example, someone undergoing vigorous chemotherapy or radiotherapy may feel sicker after treatment than at the outset of treatment. The side effects—loss of hair, loss of appetite, weakness, nausea, etc.—may make the benefits seem dubious. Hope in the possibility of overcoming these impediments is necessary to maintain the motivation to continue.[17]

Illness also challenges the more abstract or cosmic dimension of hope referred to by Marcel. Many who are seriously or chronically ill question, and even deny, a meaning to life. They lose faith in the existence of justice, Divine Providence, or beneficence in the universe. Sooner or later, Job's lament and his complaint are voiced by every seriously or chronically ill person: "Why has this happened to me?" "Why now?" "What have I done to deserve this?" These questions bespeak a loss of hope in the possibility of attaining any good at all from the experience of illness.[18] Despair leads to enervating pessimism, cynicism, and hostility. The only alternatives seem to be the defiant and scornful assertion of freedom and authenticity. Still, to sustain such defiance itself betrays a certain hope. Total despair is apt to end in requests for voluntary euthanasia or assisted suicide.

Yet properly conceived and properly employed, hope can exert a healing effect even with the dying patient.[19]

ENGENDERING HOPE

Physicians, nurses, families, friends—all who wish to help the sick person can engender or destroy hope.[20] They must nurture it in a right measure if hope is to be an aid to healing. Raising too little hope induces despair; raising too much induces false expectations. Striking this balance is an exquisitely delicate affair for which no ready formula is at hand.

Successful healing requires that the patient experience hope in the two senses described by Gabriel Marcel. We will look first at Marcel's "I hope that . . . ," i.e., the concrete hope for specific goods—in this case, health, cure, amelioration of symptoms, an easy death, etc. To undertake a course of treatment, the patient must see this as an attainable good. Physicians can give hope that the outcome will be desirable by emphasizing the successful results, the fact that dangers can be overcome, or that others have survived or had satisfactory outcomes from the same treatment.

The delicate issue is how the physician presents the information upon which hope is grounded. Every physician knows telling the truth is not enough. The physician can shape the patient's decision by the things he chooses to emphasize, omit, or include. A 25 percent chance of success, for example is statistically the same as a 75 percent chance of failure, but they sound different to the sensitized ear and emotion of a sick person.[21] The patient with hope looks to the 25 percent; the one without it, to the 75 percent. The physician who is eager to "help," or to do a particular procedure, can generate false as well as legitimate hope. Patients listen selectively when they are seriously ill. They screen out the unpleasant details and grasp, understandably, for whatever slight hope is embedded in the physician's story. The physician eager to gain experience with a new procedure or to effect a heroic result can easily delude himself or herself as well as the patient about the hope a procedure holds.[22] False hopes may arise from withholding information as much as from giving over-optimistic promises. When do we tell the quadriplegic that he will never walk again, or the juvenile diabetic what lies ahead—a shortened life and eventual kidney failure? If we reveal the whole story too soon, we rob the patient of hope that will sustain him or her in the intervening years and induce despair, which sometimes eventuates in a request for assisted suicide. If we withhold the full truth too long, we sustain the illusion of recovery, which may ultimately be shattered. If that happens, not only is hope lost but the patient also feels betrayed and loses all trust in his or her medical attendants.

This dilemma arises in any situation in which the patient suffers from a fatal, terminal, or chronically progressive disease. Physicians, out of beneficence, still invoke the "therapeutic privilege," i.e., the moral privilege of withholding information that they have grounds to believe will so rob the patient of hope that he or she will become seriously depressed or suicidal. But here too, the time will come, if the patient has not lost consciousness, when the truth will become manifest.[23]

If autonomy is to be the absolute and controlling principle in medical ethics, it favors telling the whole truth so that the patient may make his or her own choices. Those who do make autonomy an absolute principle seem willing to run the risk of despair that goes with disclosing the dire nature of one's condition.[24] Paternalists would argue, on grounds of beneficence, that the good of the patient is better served by withholding or diluting dire predictions by circumlocution. Strong paternalists would never tell the patient and would feel justified in subtle deception or lying. Weak paternalists would soften the blow by withholding information selectively and allowing the patient to grow into the realization that he or she is to die or to be permanently disabled.[25] In some cultures, it is the physician's duty to sustain hope at all costs by disclosing the truth only to family members and not to the patient.[26]

The morally appropriate choice among these alternatives and its effect on hope depend on the patient. One formula will not do for all. There are patients who will want to "know all" right away; others who will want the fullness of truth to develop slowly. At the right time, they will then ask the crucial question: "Am I going to die?" "Am I ever to walk again?" A third group may never want overtly to discuss hopelessness or face it squarely, though they may realize it privately. Finally, there are patients who will never grasp the full facts of their predicament and will persist in the illusion of recovery when it is medically futile.

Every person confronts hope and despair with his or her own unique combination of cultural, psychological, and spiritual mechanisms. We who presume to help are obliged to discern which modality best fits our patient. This is far more important than taking refuge from the difficulties by invoking some abstract principle such as autonomy, paternalistic beneficence, or therapeutic privilege. Our own preference, as we have detailed in a previous book, is to think in terms of beneficence-in-trust, i.e., acting in the best interests of the patient as defined by the patient.[27] This principle conflates autonomy into beneficence, holding that to violate autonomy is maleficence. For each patient there is an appropriate way to engender hope or prevent despair.

On this principle, for the patient who wishes to face this predicament gradually, we approach it gradually; for the patient who wants the full-strength truth right away, we lay the facts out squarely but as gently as possible. For those who wish to deny hopelessness, we take part in the drama of withholding the information but let it unfold gradually, "titrating" the patient so to speak, so that he or she can adapt to small decrements in hope, without precipitating devastating despair.[28] For the patient who hopes for a miracle, we will hope with him or her but gently allow the facts to emerge without bludgeoning the psyche with an uncompromising dose of reality.

We do not think it is morally acceptable to lie outright or to practice deception, even in the patient's interests. These things are intrinsically wrong. But they are perilous even from the pragmatic point of view. Sooner or later, the patient will discover the deception and lose all confidence in the physician. Finally, we believe the patient must eventually confront his or her predicament with its mixture of hope and despair, in order to cope with it constructively, even when death is imminent and inescapable.

The words we use to characterize engendering or dampening hope are filled with meaning. We speak of doctors "offering" no, little, or much hope or of doctors "robbing" us of hope or "holding out hope." The physician is seen as the source of hope, as if it were something he or she could dispense at will. In some ways, the physician does control the strength of hope by the words used to describe the future possibilities. To offer hope is to invite the conviction that health or cure, despite difficulties and uncertainties, will in the end be attained. This is an invitation to trust. Trust, which is central to the physician-patient relationship, is intimately united with hope. We cannot accept the offer of hope from one whom we do not trust. Correspondingly, the one who is trusted is under moral compulsion to offer only what is reasonably attainable and not to offer what is not possible.

When he or she honestly cannot offer hope the professional is suspected of robbing the patient of hope, even though the physician's interest is not to raise false hopes. The word "rob" suggests that something patients feels they own or is owed them has been illegitimately taken from them. There is a difference, therefore, between saying the doctor offered hope and saying the doctor took it away. The former bespeaks a relationship based in trust; the latter, one that is based in mistrust and hostility.

What can the physician do when there is really no hope for recovery? Can healing occur under these circumstances? What does healing mean when a patient is fatally or terminally ill? What is the good that can be offered as an object of desire and in which hope might be engendered?

If we think of healing broadly, as the reestablishment of some balance between aspirations for life and the constraints put on these aspirations by illness, then we can speak of healing even in terminally ill patients.[29] Healing in this predicament is the acceptance of living the last days of life well, i.e., of dying well. This becomes a therapeutic goal with healing power, even in the face of encroaching death. When the patient is dying, healing takes on a different meaning, but it can be attained, and hope can be engendered in its attainment, despite the obvious obstacles. This is admittedly an idiosyncratic way of looking at healing, but it is not inconsistent with the actualities of medical care.

Thus far we have discussed hope and despair as natural phenomena that health professionals and others can engender. The good hoped for is a specific good, the good of health experienced in life.

There is, as Marcel pointed out, another sense of hope—Marcel's "I hope . . ."—and to this we will turn next.

Here we confront hope in a more general sense—hope for humanity, for individual fulfillment, for meaning in life, for some transcendent good, for the world we inhabit, and for the human race. Hope must face the challenge of the universal facts of human suffering, sickness, senility, mental retardation, physical handicap, emotional distress, and human finitude. In the face of the enormous burden of their own suffering and that of others, many people lose hope in the cosmic sense. Despair undermines their faith; hope in good is displaced by hope and faith in humans or human love, or it ends in moral and spiritual nihilism. Philosophical despair has been the leitmotif of the work of Heidegger, Sartre, and Camus.[30] The pessimistic nihilism of these atheistic existentialists offers little hope to humans as individuals or as a race.

What the atheistic existentialists deny is transcendental hope, one that can go beyond the limits of what we can do for ourselves as limited human beings. While patients may not express this form of despair explicitly, it is nevertheless a subtle factor undermining recovery. Transcendental hope is much more difficult for health professionals to deal with, since its fulfillment goes beyond the technical conviction that the obstacles that stand in the way of cure or recovery from a particular illness can be overcome. If there is despair at the transcendental level (I hope . . .), there is little likelihood that hope can be engendered at the level of an actual situation (I hope that . . .).

There is little the physician can offer when the patient's healing is impeded by transcendental despair. If the physician shares the patient's cosmic pessimism, he or she may try to help by assuming Camus' or Sartre's stance. The predicament of illness can become then an occasion for an expression of existential freedom and authenticity. Like the other efforts of atheistic humanism to grapple with the mysteries of human existence, this is, at best, a temporary and rarely successful remedy.

RELIGION AND HOPE

To this point we have not dealt directly with the religious dimension of the virtue of hope. A religious perspective can address the question of hope both in its concrete and in its transcendental dimensions. Hope for Christians is one of the supernatural virtues, a habit of mind or a trait of character disposing human beings to attainment of their true end—

union with God. It grows out of acts of faith and love and is intimately intertwined with them. Hope in the Christian sense is the conviction that the *summum bonum*, the end of salvation for which humans are made, will be attained. No one is guaranteed salvation. This would be theological presumption and it would make hope unnecessary. What faith assures is the chance for salvation, that everyone will receive sufficient grace to overcome the obstacles, provided he or she does not reject the means of grace God offers in any particular circumstance.

Hope, construed as a natural virtue, is an Aristotelian mean between despair and presumption—between unwarranted pessimism and unwarranted optimism. Seen from a religious point of view, the virtue of hope disposes one to hope for fulfillment of his or her spiritual destiny. Religion deals primarily with the transcendental dimensions of hope, the "I hope . . . ," in Marcel's formulation. The religious virtue of hope is a direct denial of the absurdity of human existence as it is postulated by the atheistic existentialists or the unrelenting fatalism of the Stoics.

A faith commitment engenders hope in attaining the ultimate end of human beings. This hope is not extinguished by the predicament of illness. This is a different kind of hope from the hope that we will be cured of this disease. It is for the soul "what breathing is for the living organism. Where hope is lacking the soul dries up and withers."[31] The source of hope in this absolute sense is the Creator, to whom the creature owes existence. The creature cannot despair, since it is not in the nature of God to withdraw himself from his creation.[32] It is the presence of hope in this world that "gives meaning, rationality and genuine authenticity to man's existence here on Earth."[33]

Through this kind of hope, humans establish a relationship with God. Hope is no longer confined merely to hope for a particular outcome of a particular event in human lives. Hope transcends the impediments and even the outcomes persons may fear. It fortifies their belief that life has a purpose and that purpose is fulfilled in one's life. Illness, death, suffering, even the seemingly unjust suffering of children take on an intelligibility impossible to comprehend on natural grounds alone. This is when the theological virtue of hope appears most helpful: "There is no ultimate abandonment," it says. "You are in the lap of God."

Indeed, discovery of life's limitations and one's own propensity to disrupt the good is the basis of an individual's journey to the highest good. As MacIntyre notes:

> It is in fact this discovery of willful evil which makes the achievement of the human end possible. How? The acknowledgment by oneself of radical defect is a necessary condition for one's reception of the virtues of faith, hope, and charity. It is only the kind of knowledge which faith provides, the kind of expectation which hope provides, and the capacity for friendship with other human beings and with God which is the outcome of charity which can provide the other virtues with what they need to become genuine excellences, informing a way of life in and through which the good and the best can be achieved.[34]

We cannot expect all physicians to engender or even recognize this transcendental kind of hope. We can expect that religiously committed physicians will be aware of it in their own lives. Those who are not believers should accept its reality in the lives of their patients. Transcendental hope can be reinforced, if not by the physician, at least by spiritual and pastoral counselors. This transcendental hope is a powerful healing force, and it should be drawn upon whenever possible by those who care for the sick. Without invoking miracles, experienced clinicians know how hope in a Supreme Being who gives meaning to human life can carry patients though the most overwhelming sufferings. When health is not to be restored, this same hope leads to acceptance of death and dying. Hope sees these as occasions of healing of the soul and spirit, even if the body cannot recover. Hope robs death of despair because hope points to the story to come, which exceeds anything we can imagine on this earth.

It is surprising how frequently physicians, families, and pastoral counselors who have a faith commitment ignore the healing power of transcendental hope. There is a reluctance to draw upon the spiritual resources the patient brings to the illness or to reinforce or relight spiritual hope that has lain dormant for years. All too often physicians, pastoral counselors, and others try to help by becoming amateur (or professional) psychologists. The emotional and psychosocial dimensions of hope, healing, and despair are not to be denied. But patients need direct confrontation with the spiritual crisis they are experiencing, and psychology cannot substitute for the theological virtue of hope.

Patients in Catholic, Protestant, Jewish, and other religious hospitals, whether they are of the same persuasion as the hospital or not, rightly expect their spiritual needs to be recognized. Clearly, if patients do not wish to deal with hope in the spiritual sense, they of course have a right to reject any intrusion on their inner lives. But we must not assume that secularism has so completely permeated our society that patients must fight for a right to have their spiritual concerns legitimated every time they become ill, whether they are in secular or religiously sponsored institutions. That is not the case. We may assume the opposite in American society, in fact. Most patients would appreciate some spiritual assistance.

The obligation to provide such assistance applies to physicians who are nonbelievers as well as to believers. All physicians can engender hope or despair by the very fact of their entry into the patient's predicament of illness. The nonbeliever is under no compulsion to change his or her own point of view, but only to recognize that healing, "making whole," as the etymology of the word indicates, requires an extension of the healer into the spirit as well as the body of the sick person. By nature, human beings are spiritual as well as physical entities, and they cannot be healed without attending to their spiritual needs.

Indeed, much of the despair—and a considerable part of the suffering—patients endure in the face of incurable illness today is the result of a loss of transcendental hope, even among believers. Surely the growing trend in favor of euthanasia and assisted suicide is fired in significant measure by a loss of hope. The resultant despair and despondency lead to a desire for death by any means. As a result, "compassion" is redefined as assisting the patient to enter oblivion. This is false compassion.[35] True compassion would require entering into the experience of suffering, and helping the patient to regain transcendental hope, a much more challenging and even threatening enterprise. In this way, patients grow spiritually just when the physical body has reached its point of exhaustion.

The Christian virtue of hope is essential, therefore, for healing to take place—healing of the body and the mind and the soul. Hope in God's design for us, in his mercy, and in his promise of an afterlife whose glories we cannot even conceive provides the motivation to sustain and relieve our suffering even when death is inevitable. Christian hope is essential for the doctor as well as the patient. The doctor, too, must hope, in the transcendental sense defined by Marcel. That hope will enable him or her to endure amid the daily round of suffering, depressed, and even despairing humans it is the doctor's privilege to treat.

Christian hope is, however, not a simple, romantic disavowal of the reality of suffering and dying. It does not require replacing the benefits of medical care, however limited they may be in some cases, with pious presumption that a miracle will occur. Christian hope recognizes that God may, indeed, work a miracle, but it also recognizes that his goodness and solicitude are there regardless of whether a miracle occurs. Sometimes the bedside becomes a battleground where families almost seem to dare God or coerce him into supplying a miracle. Christian hope is not an invitation to unrealism or false expectations. It confronts the realities of the patient's predicament, but it directs the mind and heart to something much larger, the reality of God's presence in history, his promises to humanity, and his unfailing love for every one of his creatures.

CONCLUSION: WHY ME?

Individuals have a choice. They may take as a model Job or Sisyphus. Both were the subjects of intense suffering in which hope, both concrete and cosmic, appeared to be gone from their lives. Job found out through long dialogues with his well-meaning but wrong-headed friends that his sufferings were not the result of sin. Job learned that he had no claim on God, that he had to hope even though he seemed robbed of the hope that arises in the knowledge of God's love for us. Job found out, finally, that there would be no explanation that he could understand, that he had to hope in God's justice, and in the end he found that by surrendering his will he was restored.

Sisyphus, on the other hand, was condemned to his unending rock, rolling it up to the top of the hill and down again, because he practiced deception. He had, unlike Job, sinned by attempting to deceive the gods. He really did not have any basis for hope. His gods were capable of abandoning him, and they did indeed do so.

Whether we see hope as Job did, his protests notwithstanding, or as Sisyphus did depends upon whether we believe we are created beings in whom the Creator continues to have interest or whether we are pagans whose gods have no commitment to humans, only hegemony over them. As Thomas Merton, with his usual lucidity and conciseness puts it, "He who hopes in God trusts in God, Whom he never sees, to bring him in possession of things that are beyond imagination."[36] Moreover, hope completes the other virtues of faith and love: "Without hope, our faith gives us only an acquaintance with God. Without love and hope, faith only knows Him as a stranger."[37] Thus, hope impels us to use whatever means God has put at our disposal in the pursuit of our lives. This is so because hope assures us that what natural gifts we have can be elevated by grace in such a way that we achieve what, by our natural perceptions, we think beyond us.

These perceptions of hope are relevant to the patient's predicament of illness and the physician's act of healing. They embolden patient and physician to use what natural powers they possess and what human science affords them. But hope also means that if these measures fail, as too often they do, all is not lost; God's love will bring us into possessions "beyond imagination."

NOTES

1. Translation from "Chapter 8: The Mutual Dependence of Hope and Love," in *The Works of Aurelius Augustinus, Bishop of Hippo (Being a Treatise on Faith, Hope, and Love)*, ed. and trans. Martin Dods (Edinburgh: T. and T. Clark, 1873).

2. William F. Lynch, *Images of Hope* (Baltimore: Helicon Books, 1965), pp. 31–34.

3. St. Thomas Aquinas, *Summa Theologiae* [Vol. 22], ed. Anthony Kenny (New York: Blackfriars, 1964), I-II, q. 50, a. 5, pp. 42–45.

4. Virgil, *The Aeneid*, trans. J. W. Mackail (Oxford: Clarendon Press, 1930), p. 419.

5. Sr. Madeleine Clemence Vaillot, "Living and Dying, Part I: Hope, the Restoration of Being," *American Journal of Nursing* 70, no. 2 (1970): 268–272.

6. Jan S. Schneider, "Hopelessness and Helplessness," *Journal of Practical Nursing and Mental Health Services* 18, no. 3 (1980): 12–21.

7. Susan Baird, "Why Hope Now?" *Oncology Nursing Forum* 16, no. 1 (1989): 9.

8. Gabriel Marcel, *Fresh Hope for the World* (London: Longmans, 1960).

9. Albert Camus, *"The Myth of Sisyphus" and Other Essays*, trans. Justin O'Brien (New York: Knopf, 1955).

10. Robert M. Green, trans., *A Translation of Galen's Hygiene (De Sanitate Tuenda)* (Springfield, Ill.: Thomas, 1951), bk. 1, p. 5.

11. Jurrit Bergsma and David C. Thomasma, *Healthcare: Its Psychosocial Dimensions* (Pittsburgh: Duquesne University Press, 1982).

12. Eric J. Cassell, "The Function of Medicine," *Hastings Center Report* 7, no. 6 (1977): 16–19.

13. Mary L. Nowotny, "Assessment of Hope in Patients with Cancer: Development of an Instrument," *Oncology Nursing Forum* 16, no. 1 (1989): 57–79.

14. Arthur H. Schmale and Howard P. Iker, "The Affect of Hopelessness and the Development of Cancer," *Psychosomatic Medicine* 28, no. 8 (1966): 714–721.

15. I. N. Korner, "Hope as a Method of Coping," *Journal of Consulting and Clinical Psychology* 34, no. 2 (1970): 134–139.

16. Richard T. Roessler and Susan E. Boone, "The Paradox of Hope for Individuals with a Disability," *Psychosocial Rehabilitation Journal* 2, no. 1 (1978): 1–8.

17. Kaye A. Herth notes that studies demonstrate that hope and coping are intimately related ("The Relationship between Level of Hope and Level of Coping Response and Other Variables in Patients with Cancer," *Oncology Nursing Forum* 16, no. 1 [1989]: 67–79). See also S. Greer, T. Morris, and K. W. Pettingale, "Psychological Response to Breast Cancer: Effect on Outcome," *Lancet* 2, no. 8146 (1979): 785–787.

18. Near the end of the first millennium of Christianity, Pope St. Gregory the Great offered replies to Job's questions, based on the revelation in the New Testament. His interest in the questions was prompted by the human condition of illness and suffering in his own day. Moreover, the entirety of Scripture can be read as a struggle to explain the problem of evil. Commenting on John 18:36, "My kingdom is not of this world," St. Gregory says, "All we then who being embued with the hope of heaven wear ourselves out with the toiling of the present life, are busiest in the concern of another." See St. Gregory the Great, *Morals on the Book of Job* [Vol. 1] (Oxford: John Henry Parker, 1844), bk. 7, 1.12, p. 422.

19. Kevin A. Kraus, "Hoping in the Healing Process: An Integral Condition to the Ethics of Care." Doctoral dissertation, Washington, Georgetown University, 1993.

20. Judith F. Miller, "Inspiring Hope," *American Journal of Nursing* 85, no. 1 (1985): 22–25.

21. David C. Thomasma, "Decision-Making and Decision Analysis: Beneficence in Medicine," *Journal of Critical Care* 3, no. 2 (1988): 122–132.

22. David C. Thomasma, "When Healing Involves Risk to Life: Risky Medical Procedures and Experimentation," *New Catholic World* 230 (July/August, 1987): 163–167.

23. Dennis Novack *et al.*, "Physicians' Attitudes toward Using Deception to Resolve Difficult Ethical Problems," *Journal of the American Medical Association* 261, no. 20 (1989): 2980–2985.

24. This problem also applies to knowing ahead of time one's own or one's children's genetic makeup. Joseph F. Fletcher suggests that some knowledge may not be good to know (*The Ethics of Genetic Control* [Buffalo: Prometheus Books, 1988]).

25. See the discussion of these approaches in Charles Culver and Bernard Gert, *Philosophy in Medicine: Conceptual and Ethical Issues in Medicine and Psychiatry* (New York: Oxford University Press, 1982), pp. 126–163; Rose F. McGee, "Hope: A Factor Influencing Crisis Resolution," *Advances in Nursing Science* 6, no. 4 (1984): 34–44.

26. Antonella Surbone, "Truth Telling to the Patient," *Journal of the American Medical Association* 268, no. 13 (1992): 1661–1662.

27. Edmund D. Pellegrino and David C. Thomasma, *For the Patient's Good: Toward the Restoration of Beneficence in Health Care* (New York: Oxford University Press, 1988).

28. E. Rideout and M. Montemuro, "Hope, Morale, and Adaptation in Patients with Chronic Heart Failure," *Journal of Advanced Nursing* 11, no. 4 (1986): 429–438.

29. If hope is to be seen as an action concept, a method of coping, then continuing to hope is a way of healing oneself. See also Howard Brody, "Sickness and Self-Respect," in *Stories of Sickness* (London: Yale University Press, 1987), pp. 41–58.

30. Martin Heidegger, *The Question of Technology and Other Essays*, trans. William Lovitt (New York: Harper and Row, 1977); Jean Paul Sartre, *Nausea*, trans. Lloyd Alexander (New York: New Directions, 1964); Camus, *"Myth of Sisyphus" and Other Essays*.

31. Gabriel Marcel, *Homo Viator* (New York: Henry Regnery, 1951), pp. 10–11.

32. Marcel, *Homo Viator*, pp. 46–47.

33. Francis J. Lescoe, *Existentialism: With or without God* (New York: Alba House, 1974), p. 114.

34. Alasdair MacIntyre, *Three Rival Versions of Moral Enquiry: Encyclopedia, Genealogy, and Tradition* (Notre Dame: University of Notre Dame Press, 1990), p. 140.

35. Edmund D. Pellegrino, "Compassion Needs Reason Too," *Journal of the American Medical Association* 270, no. 7 (1993): 874–875.

36. Thomas Merton, *No Man Is an Island* (New York: Harcourt, Brace, 1955), p. 15.

37. Merton, *No Man Is an Island*, p. 16.

5

Charity: The Ordering Principle of Christian Ethics

In any religious ethics of medicine, charity is the ordering principle of all the other virtues.[1] In this sense, Christian ethics is a love-inspired ethics, i.e., an agapeistic ethic. Charity unifies every act under an obligation that transcends ordinary duties.[2] Denis J. B. Hawkins puts it well: "What is distinctive of the moral teaching of the gospel is not a new code of morality or a new theory of its basis, but the insistence on raising morality to the level of love. The commandments are to find their full meaning and completion in the love of God and our neighbor for God's sake."[3]

This is what St. Thomas teaches when he makes charity the "form" of the virtues.[4] Gerard Gilleman provides a particularly compelling account of Thomistic teaching on this point. He shows how charity gives every virtuous act and, indeed, every virtue a supernatural moral worth by orienting each to its final end, which, for the theological virtues, is a supernatural one, i.e., union with God.[5] An ethic shaped according to the virtue of charity is an agapeistic ethic, an ethic that goes beyond principle, rule, or obligation not by absorbing or negating but by perfecting it in a way no moral syllogism possibly could.

For the religious physician, therefore, the moral life is conducted from several perspectives not shared by nonbelievers, e.g., the perspectives of creatureliness and incarnation.[6] As a result, one's natural tendencies and purposes are measured against a larger purpose of human life, and the Creator's purposes. In this view, human beings are expected and enabled to go "beyond the possibilities of nature left to itself."[7]

Clearly, in a Christian ethic, the motivation for being moral is explicitly different from what it is in a naturalistic ethic. The Christian knows that doing the right and the good is a means of growing closer to God the Creator and Redeemer. The believer also has in charity an ordering principle that illuminates a central dilemma of philosophical ethics: why, and to what degree, are some rules and principles morally imperative and others not, and which among the possible sources of morality should take precedence? In conformity to God's will, as John Crosby argues, a believer recognizes that "the binding force of moral obligation ultimately derives from divine command."[8]

This entails more than fulfilling duty in response to a reasoned argument about what ought to be done. Instead, the encounter with God in moral choice demands that the end of a religious person's reasoned judgment must be a right attitude of mind and heart. The virtue of charity, therefore, consists in disposing moral judgments to their right end through love for God and the human family He has created. Charity fuses the qualities of both mind and heart, of reason and faith—a fusion without meaning in a nonagapeistic ethic.

MEDICAL PRACTICE AND CHARITY: WHAT DIFFERENCE DOES CHARITY MAKE?

If there is something distinctive about an ethic based in the virtue of charity, it ought to be manifest in practical moral decisions. Medicine is a praxis, an activity with its own internal goal. Fidelity to that goal—the good of the patient—is a moral obligation. An agapeistic perspective should therefore dispose the physician to decisions that would advance the good of the patient, but in a way informed by charity.

To be able to make choices consistent with the virtue of charity requires a particular orientation of the capacity for deliberation in the Aristotelian sense. This capacity, when shaped by a religious perspective, should dispose the believing physician to select among the many particulars of a concrete moral choice those which most closely conform to the virtue of charity. This entails a special kind of phronesis, a practical wisdom oriented and motivated by the virtue of charity to act in a way pleasing to the Divinity, as perceived in any particular situation.

Three aspects of medical moral decisions will serve to illustrate how the Christian virtue of charity shapes moral choice: (1) the way the dominant principles of medical ethics are interpreted; (2) the way the physician-patient relationship is construed; and (3) the way certain concrete choices in contemporary professional ethics are made.

1. Charity and the Principles of Ethics

An agapeistic ethic is by definition a virtue-based ethic. It must confront, therefore, the dilemma of how virtue relates to rules, duties, and principles. This is a prickly problem for any comprehensive philosophy of the moral life, as we have explored elsewhere.[9] The problem is particularly relevant for Christian ethics, for, as Anthony Ple points out, "it is not possible to love out of duty, that is, solely for the reason that authority imposes upon me the obligation of loving."[10] To recognize this fact is not to agree with Ple's full indictment of the morality of duty as an "obsessional neurosis" or with the primarily psychologistic line of his argument.

Principles, rules, and duties are as much a reality of the moral life as love and cannot be fully disengaged from it. What may be the essential difference in an agapeistic ethic is that rules, duties, and principles are chosen—or shaped—by charity, i.e., by whether they foster its growth, a fact even Ple admits.[11]

The primary principles of medical ethics—beneficence, justice, and autonomy—are ascertainable by human reason without resort to the revelation of Sacred Scripture. For some, they are prima facie principles, intuitively perceived.[12] As such, they enjoy widespread acceptance today even in our morally pluralistic society. They can be expanded by religious belief, not contracted and reduced. What the virtue of charity adds is a special way in which these principles are to be lived and applied in concrete situations. In a religious perspective, charity "informs" these principles. When prima facie principles conflict, charity sorts out resolutions that are in the spirit of the Beatitudes from those that are not. This spirit lies in the personhood of Jesus himself such that the resolutions conform not only to the many dimensions of peaceable community life but also to God drawing us personally toward Himself in love.

Each of the principles of medical ethics is thus subject to tests of conformity with normative sources of moral validation—Scripture, the tradition or teaching of an official church, the example of Jesus—not acknowledged by the nonbeliever. As a result, a Christian ethic of medicine imposes levels of obligation that, on purely naturalist grounds, are optional or supererogatory. For example, the Christian is exhorted unequivocally to perfection in charity by the Sermon on the Mount. On reason alone such a pursuit could be accounted as unreasonable, unrealistic, psychologically unattainable, or guilt-producing.

Beneficence—acting for the good of the patient—is the central principle of medical ethics. But beneficence is interpretable at several levels, from mere nonmaleficence to heroic sacrifice. Health professionals may differ sharply on precisely what degree of beneficence they consider binding. Some argue that not harming the patient is sufficient, invoking the oft-quoted principle "Primum non nocere." Others feel bound to a more positive interpretation—i.e., acting for the good of the patient, not just avoiding harm—thus injecting some degree of altruism. Still others feel impelled to benevolent self-effacement—that is to say, acting for the patient's good even if it means doing so at some personal cost in time, convenience, danger to self, or financial loss. Finally, for a very few, such as Mother Teresa, or Father Damien with the lepers, beneficence means heroic sacrifices and complete dedication to the needs of the sick and dying. This degree of self-sacrifice closely approximates the degree of perfection that perfect charity would require and that Jesus himself demonstrated. Thus, St. Francis was repelled by lepers and shunned them like most in society until he was impelled to embrace them from the love of Christ. A comparison to attitudes toward patients with AIDS is inescapable. Few can be expected to attain this degree of beneficence, but it remains an ideal toward which a Christian should strive with the limits of grace open to him or her.

From this perspective, however, benevolent self-effacement is a minimum obligation consistent with the virtue of charity. Lesser degrees of the virtue of benevolence and beneficence would be inconsistent with such scriptural exhortations as the story of the Good Samaritan and the Sermon on the Mount and with Jesus' own healing acts. On this view medical knowledge is not proprietary or simply a means to a living. It is a means of service to others, a mission and apostolate, a ministry to those who have a special claim on the whole community—the especially vulnerable, the sick, disabled, poor, or retarded.[13] Meeting the claims of the vulnerable is an essential feature of Christian belief. It is not optional or heroic. The healing ministry of the church is not an appendage through which compassion is titrated. It is the presence of Christ in the world.

Thus, for a religious person, the practice of medicine is a moral calling. It is transformed from a mere occupation or profession to a vocation, a call from God to a specific way of gaining one's own salvation and assisting others to their salvation. Practicing medicine as a Christian requires giving witness to the truth of the faith in the way one lives his or her personal and professional life. Medicine seen as a vocation becomes a way to spiritualize our own lives and those of others.

When it is practiced in accord with charity as its ordering principle, medicine takes on levels of meaning that transcend even the nobler traditions of the profession secularly conceived. Those who do not share the convictions of the Christian often attain high degrees of self-effacement in the service of the sick. This should challenge religiously committed caregivers even more. The Christian is called to a degree of perfection of his or her practice that extends from the intent to the performance of all professional acts in conformity with the virtue of charity. Each is counseled, "You therefore are to be perfect even as your Heavenly Father is perfect" (Matthew 5:48).

What does this mean in practical terms? Does it somehow make the Christian a superior being just by virtue of his or her belief? Does it make his or her acts ipso facto morally superior? Does it demean the dedication, commitment, and genuine love of nonbelievers who care sincerely and with affection and love for the sick? Certainly not.

Nor does it mean that the Christian physician can ever fully achieve conformity with an ineffable model of the healer.[14] That healer is Jesus Christ, whose love for the afflicted was completely free of selfish interest. It had only the good of the sick as its end, completely freed from any taint of self-satisfaction. Solicitous healing of the lame came to Jesus as an expression of his and the Father's love for all humans, good and bad, agreeable and disagreeable, clean and dirty, rich and poor, grateful and ungrateful. Unlike the natural virtue of benevolence, Jesus' charity asked nothing in return; its effacement of self-interest was complete.

Can we fairly expect this of even the committed believer? We know, of course, that such perfection is not attainable by even the most perfect of humans, but we are required to strive for it, and to understand that, unlike the nonbeliever, we cannot be faithful to our belief without living it to the fullest extent possible, that if we are charitable, it is because we have accepted the grace necessary, and that this grace had God as its source. Indeed, in ways we cannot discern, God's grace is present in the charitable acts of nonbelievers as well.

Thus, the Christian physician must strive for perfection in the natural ends of medical healing but also in its supernatural ends. It is in the constant awareness and effort to respond to these ends and their fusion that grace perfects nature. Perfect charity is, therefore, not a duty or obligation, because it cannot be a supernatural virtue unless it is freely chosen out of a pure intention that seeks the good of the other person for its own sake. It allows the other person also to be free, to be helped even if he chooses not to be like me and, indeed, resists being like me or conforming to my notion of what is good for him.

Thus, charity respects the autonomy of the patient in a way different than autonomy is respected in a purely naturally conceived formulation of the principle. Charity cannot be possessive, self-congratulating, or self-righteous. If it is, it is not perfect charity, whether it is a Christian or a non-Christian who practices it. If medicine is accepted by us as a Christian vocation, then God wills it not because we like it, nor because it satisfies us, but because it is the way God wants us to use the talents he has given us. To follow our vocations with true charity, we must strive earnestly to act for the sick, to advocate their cause, and, when their interests require it, to expose ourselves to the dangers of infection, inconvenience, the invasion of private time, financial sacrifice, and ingratitude. Rudeness, inaccessibility, abruptness, refusal to treat for economic reasons, discrimination because of social class, ethnicity, etc., are not reconcilable with a charity-based ethic of medicine; neither is medicine practiced as a business, an exercise in entrepreneurship, as applied biology, politics, or societal convenience.[15]

Charity provides no algebraic formula measuring out the degree of effacement of self-interest that one must practice in a specific situation. Nor does it provide a precise line that can divide legitimate self-interest from the requirement of self-effacement. The virtue of charity also calls for proper care of self and of one's familial, social, and communal relationships, all of which also require love and concern for others. What is clear is that an agapeistic ethic accepts no easy justification for reducing beneficence to mere nonmaleficence, autonomy to either paternalism or absolute subjection to the patient's will, or justice to legalistic compliance with a contract.

An agapeistic ethic calls the physician to perfection in charity even though he or she cannot succeed entirely, given the ineffability of Christ, of the model he or she must emulate. That believing physicians and other health professionals do, in fact, fall short of the benevolent self-effacement charity requires is obvious. But they should know when they have fallen short. They should strive to come closer always, not as an act of noble self-sacrifice but as an obedient response to a loving God (Luke 6:36).[16] Every argument from exigency, fiscal survival, or conformity to the prevailing mores must be scrutinized from this perspective.

A religious ethics' view of compassion, then, mitigates the conflict bioethics scholars may see between the principles of beneficence and autonomy by linking duties we have to others with the promotion of their own well-being. Quite obviously such a perspective shapes the way we interpret and apply the principles of medical ethics in specific ways. Nonbelievers may interpret them the same way, but they need not do so. If they do, they use different reasons. More is rightly expected of those who profess to emulate the example of Jesus' healing. For them the obligations to respect autonomy, justice, and beneficence are at the service of charity. These principles gain their worth not aprioristically but because they express what is necessary to the virtue of charity. Indeed, true charity embraces all of these principles and gives them a single motivation, that of love.

Whether this perspective calls for supererogation if examined on purely philosophical grounds is problematic. The status of supererogation in moral theory—whether it is a separate category or encompassable in Kantian deontology—is still a debatable question.[17] All we need to say at this point is that the range of interpretations of philosophical ethical principles and duties is specified in particular ways in a charity-based ethic.

There are some problem areas, however. Respect for the inviolability of human conscience may bring the believing physician or nurse into moral conflict with the autonomous decisions of patients, families, other health professionals, the hospital, and even the state. In a charity-based ethics, the professional is obliged to handle the conflict with love and respect for those with whom he or she disagrees. But on the same principle, the health professional cannot cooperate formally or directly with an intrinsically evil act. There is the obligation to decide whether to withdraw respectfully or, if the harm being done—e.g., active euthanasia, grossly incompetent surgery—is sufficiently great, to intervene directly. One may use those means available in democratic societies—persuasion, ethics committees, and the courts—but not violent means, which violate the virtue of charity.

A charity-based ethics cannot uncritically accept the current move from substantive to procedural ethics. Such a move is useful and doubtless necessary in a morally pluralistic society. Nonetheless, even in the interests of amicable settlement of moral conflicts, the substance of moral decisions must be defended. This means that a certain tension will exist between secular and Christian ethics in such matters as pre-embryo experimentation, fertilization of fetal ova, or surrogate motherhood, for example. Likewise, these substantive ethical issues are not truly resolved if professional ethical codes are revised to fit the needs of morally pluralistic societies. This has already happened with abortion and is likely to occur with euthanasia.

2. Christian Charity and Professional Practices

If we move from principles to concrete moral dilemmas, we can perhaps see more clearly how charity acts as a principle of discernment and how it orders some of the moral decisions facing health professionals today. We can use as illustrations a few professional practices that have not been declared immoral by the profession as a whole and that are even accepted, however reluctantly, on grounds of necessity or economic survival. We refer here to a range of practices—some old, some new—that compromise, endanger, or conflict with the best interests of patients. Examples include working in for-profit managed health care systems and medical entrepreneurship in its many forms—investing in and owning health care facilities to which one refers patients, misleading advertising, selling and dispensing medication, refusing to see Medicare or Medicaid patients, charging excessive fees, gatekeeping in its various forms, pay-as-you-go research,[18] cutting corners to contain costs or enhance profits, the many marketing artifices that ensure success in competition and the marketplace, etc. This list of morally marginal practices is spawned by the current commercialization and monetarization of health care as an industry that legitimates the financial motivations of health professionals, administrators, and owners of health care facilities.

These practices are justified on "practical" or economic grounds as means to cost containment and managerial efficiency. Many consider them salubrious to the general welfare so long as provisions are made to avoid abuses. Even Catholic and other religiously sponsored hospitals and health professionals are all too enthusiastically embracing some of these practices in the name of exigency. They are at the heart of the present debate about health care reform.

It is difficult to justify such practices in any truly agapeistic ethic. The possibilities that the patient's interest will be submerged by the financial interests of the health professional or institution and medicine downgraded from a vocation to a business are all too obvious. Many of these practices have been condemned repeatedly as morally dubious even on nonreligious grounds. How much more reprehensible are they when practiced by physicians and institutions that lay claim to the title "Christian"? It is often in the realm of the morally marginal, rather than the frankly immoral, that the more stringent requirements of an agapeistic ethic are most easily discerned.

Today many religious physicians, nurses, administrators, and hospitals justify their compromising the virtue of charity on grounds of exigency and survival. Thus, they give proof to the mordant observation of Machiavelli that "a man who wishes to act entirely up to his professions of virtue soon meets with what destroys him among so much that is evil."[19] But is it not the challenge of Christian ethics to do precisely what Machiavelli thought impossible?

CHARITY AND THE PHYSICIAN-PATIENT RELATIONSHIP

Similarly, adherence to a Christian and charity-based ethic shapes the model of the physician- or nurse-patient relationship. Certain of the models now being proposed become morally distasteful, if not totally unacceptable. Thus, a genuine Christian ethic would be incompatible with health care as a commodity transaction and the healing relationship as a commercial activity. The idea of the physician as primarily a businessperson is inconsistent with the Christian ethic of medicine. Likewise, such an ethic would reject the healing relationship as primarily an exercise in applied biology or as a legal contract for services. Nor could the relationship be construed as paternalistic, or as primarily a means of livelihood, personal profit, or prestige for the physician. Equally incompatible are models that make the physician primarily a government bureaucrat, a proletarian employee of a corporation, or an agent of the state as in totalitarian regimes.

Instead, the model of physician-patient relationships most consistent with a Christian ethic is the covenant, in which the physician pledges fidelity to a binding promise to help.[20] That promise does not call for total, unquestioning submission to the good as defined by the patient but to the higher levels of charitable beneficence alluded to earlier. On the Christian view, the idea of a profession embraces the higher ideals of a commitment to service subsumed in the idea of a Christian vocation.[21]

Parenthetically, a religious conception of the healing relationship imposes certain obligations on the patients as well. Honesty, compliance with the doctor's regimen, refraining from frivolous, frankly unjust, or injurious legal action, and respect for the humanity and moral values of the physician are logical corollaries of a covenantal relationship. A shared respect by Christian physician and patient for the virtue of charity therefore is essential.

The physician-patient relationship—and equally the nurse-, dentist-, and pharmacist-patient relationships—does not, however, call for a monastic devotion to medicine to the exclusion of other obligations to family, self, society, or country. It does not deny the fact that in some measure medicine is simultaneously a business, a craft, a science, and a technology. But what an agapeistic ethics does preeminently is to place these differing facets of medical practice into a morally defensible order, recognizing when, and to what degree, they must yield to the ordering principle of charity.

This is essentially what it means to say that charity is the form of the virtues. Charity acts as a practical principle of discernment and a benchmark against which the Christian measures concretely, here and now, the moral worth of his or her practical decisions. Often it is said that the Scriptures give no categorical guidance, no set rules for resolving all the dilemmas of medical ethics. Apart from the Beatitudes, this is so. Manifestly, the Scriptures could not anticipate every possible moral dilemma that might arise in the history of humanity. But they add something more valuable. They teach that charity is the form of all the virtues, that charity is the ordering principle of discernment in moral choice. And they are very specific in detailing what charity comprises—all the concrete examples in Jesus' own life, what he meant in concrete situations by the transcendental ethos of charity, which he preached and taught on the Mount in full view of the needy of all the world.

The health professional and institution that profess Christianity must heed that Sermon every day in every encounter with the sick. It is in this sense that the Christian perspective sees through and beyond philosophical medical ethics to the virtue of charity. Charity becomes an interior principle, as it were, that encompasses the philosophically derivable internal morality of medicine and, without abrogating it, transmutes healing into an act of grace.

CONCLUSION

What we have tried to show is the way adherence to Christian belief and teaching is based in the virtue of charity. We do not mean to suggest that Christian health care professionals do, in fact, uniformly practice their professions in a spirit of true charity or that by that fact they are morally superior to non-Christians or nonbelievers. Indeed, all too frequently, Christians fail in the virtue of charity or are exceeded in the practice of the natural virtues by those who do not accept, or reject outright, the virtue of charity as it is portrayed in the Gospels. Our principal aim has been to show what is required of Christians who hope to be faithful to the faith they espouse and what difference this should make in how they practice medicine.

This is not an invitation to complacency or pious self-righteousness but an admonition. A profession of Christian faith is a declaration of intent to act charitably, and any failure to do so is a failure of commitment to a promise and, therefore, is an act of infidelity and hypocrisy. This should become more apparent in the following chapters, which detail the way charity transforms the usual principles of medical ethics.

NOTES

1. Henry Bars, *Faith, Hope, and Charity,* trans. P. J. Hepburne Scott (New York: Hawthorne Books, 1961); Denis J. B. Hawkins, *Christian Ethics,* vol. 8 of *The Twentieth Century Encyclopedia of Catholicism,* ed. Henri Daniel-Rops (New York: Hawthorne Books, 1963), pp. 1–125; St. Augustine, *Faith, Hope, and Charity,* trans. L. Arand (New York: Newman Bookshop, 1947); St. Augustine, *The Lord's Sermon on the Mount,* trans. J. Jepson (Westminster, Md.: Newman Press, 1948).

2. *Catechism of the Catholic Church* (Mahwah, N.J.: Paulist Press, 1994), pt. 3, sec. 2, chap. 1, art. 1 and 2, pp. 505–522; and sec. 1, chap. 1, art. 7, no. 2, pp. 446–450.

3. Hawkins, *Christian Ethics,* p. 28.

4. St. Thomas Aquinas, *Summa Theologiae* [Vol. 34], ed. and trans. R. J. Batten (New York: Blackfriars, 1975), II-II, q. 23, a. 8, pp. 30–33.

5. Gerard Gilleman, *The Primacy of Charity in Moral Theology* (Westminster, Md.: Newman Press, 1959), p. 53.

6. Hawkins, *Christian Ethics,* p. 16.

7. Hawkins, *Christian Ethics,* pp. 16–17.

8. John F. Crosby, "The Encounter of God and Man in Moral Obligation," *New Scholasticism* 60, no. 3 (1986): 317–355 at 317.

9. Edmund D. Pellegrino and David C. Thomasma, *The Virtues in Medicine* (New York: Oxford University Press, 1993), pp. 18–30.

10. Anthony Ple, "The Morality of Duty and Obsessional Neurosis," *Cross Currents* 36, no. 3 (1986): 343–357.

11. Ple, "Morality of Duty," p. 344.

12. Tom L. Beauchamp and James F. Childress, *Principles of Bioethics,* 3d ed. (New York: Oxford University Press, 1989).

13. Pope John Paul II, *Apostolic Letter: Salvifici Doloris* (Washington: U.S. Catholic Conference, 1984).

14. Thomas Merton, *No Man Is an Island* (New York: Harcourt, Brace, 1955), pp. 165–169.

15. David C. Thomasma, "Entrepreneurship in Medicine," in *Health Care Ethics: Critical Issues*, ed. J. F. Monagle and D. C. Thomasma (Rockville, Md.: Aspen Publications, 1994), pp. 342–349.

16. Donald P. McNeill, Douglas A. Morrison, and Henri Nouwen, eds., *Compassion: A Reflection on the Christian Life* (New York: Doubleday, 1982).

17. Marcia Baron, "Kantian Ethics and Supererogation," *Journal of Philosophy* 84, no. 5 (1987): 237–262.

18. Julia M. Reade and Richard M. Ratzan, "Yellow Professionalism: Advertising by Physicians in the Yellow Pages," *New England Journal of Medicine* 316, no. 21 (1987): 1315–1319; Arnold S. Relman, "Practicing Medicine in the New Business Climate," *New England Journal of Medicine* 316, no. 18 (1987): 1150–1151.

19. Nicolo Machiavelli, *The Prince* [Great Books, vol. 22] (Chicago: Encyclopedia Britannica, 1952), p. 22.

20. William F. May, *The Physician's Covenant* (Philadelphia: Westminster Press, 1983); Edmund D. Pellegrino and David C. Thomasma, *For the Patient's Good: The Restoration of Beneficence in Health Care* (New York: Oxford University Press, 1988).

21. Edmund D. Pellegrino, "Professional Ethics: Moral Decline or Paradigm Shift?" *Religion and Intellectual Life* 4, no. 3 (1987): 21–39.

6

Charity in Action: Compassion and Caring

> *Before all, and above all, attention should be paid to the care of the sick so that they shall be served as if they were Christ himself.*
>
> —Rule of St. Benedict

> *The only difference between kindness and benevolence is that one is exterior while the other is interior; kindness being merely benevolence carried into effect. Accordingly, just as benevolence is not another virtue distinct from charity, so also kindness.*
>
> — St. Thomas Aquinas[1]

Every Christian will readily agree that the sick person is his sister or brother. After all, are we not all sons and daughters of the same Father? But as in our immediate families, so in the human family, the sick person is brother or sister in a special way. The one who is sick has a special claim on our solicitude, love, and compassion, for without meeting these claims, the healer cannot truly heal.

JESUS' CALL TO HEALING

Jesus gave us the most compelling examples of the special solicitude we should show the sick. Healing filled his daily life. He was always among the suffering. Half of Mark's Gospel, perhaps the earliest account of the Lord's mission to the infirm, is devoted to narratives of healing. In Luke he teaches us by the parable of the Good Samaritan that the stranger is our neighbor who deserves not only our love but also our sacrifice. For Jesus, healing the sick was intrinsic to his salvific mission. And so, too, it must be for those who profess to be his followers.

One of the most beautiful evocations of Christ's compassion for the sick is the depiction in the first chapter of Mark: "Now when it was evening and the sun had set they brought unto him all who were ill and who were possessed. And the whole town gathered at the door. And he cured many who were afflicted with various diseases and cast out many devils."[2] This is a scene repeated many times over. Wherever he went, tired, dusty from the road, pressed in upon by human needs of all kinds, Jesus always had time for the sick, the disabled, and the handicapped.

The Gospels also teach another lesson: concern for the sick and their healing involves the whole community. It was their families and friends who brought the halt, the blind, and the deaf to Jesus. It was they who begged his help insistently. At Capernaum, they even dismantled the roof to lower a paralytic into his presence. Christ's healing itself was a community affair. He healed in public, with family and friends looking on and sharing the experience.

We who profess to be Christians are committed to emulate Christ's example. As individuals and communities, we are called to "put on Christ" (Galatians 3:27), to see the sick as he saw them, to make the healing ministry a part of our lives.

SICKNESS IN TODAY'S WORLD

What does this mean in our times, which are different in so many ways from Jesus' time? In our world the sick are often removed from our immediate presence to the hospital, hospice, or nursing home. Their care is assigned to strangers and professionals. They suffer and die surrounded by the apparatus of technology, often unable to communicate their needs. Their friends and families live at a distance. It is hard for friends and family to be present to the sick in their moments of greatest need.

Our attitudes toward sickness have changed drastically. In Jesus' time, sickness and death were inescapable conditions of human existence over which there was little hope of rational control. Today, sickness has become a scandal, a contradiction to our technological hubris and frenetic pursuit of the cult of health, youth, and pleasure. We routinely expect medical miracles to exorcise illness. But the sick person is a brutal reminder of the finitude and frailty we want so much to deny.

Rather than being our brothers and sisters, the sick have become alien to us—inhabitants of a world that is not ours, a world we hope (however unrealistically) we will never occupy.

The response of the Christian community is vastly different, too. Traditionally, we had thought of care of the sick as a social need far distant from the values of the marketplace. To heal was a work of mercy, not a commodity to be traded or delivered. Now we worry instead about the resources the sick divert from our other projects. We talk of rationing the care we give, especially to the most vulnerable among us—the poor, the elderly, the chronically handicapped, the infants, the mentally ill, and the retarded. We shrink from the sacrifice—of our time, emotions, energies, and money—that the care of the sick so much requires. So urgent has the economics of health care become that some religious orders and dioceses even contemplate withdrawing from this vital ministry. The statistical morality of the macroeconomists is overshadowing the virtue of Christian charity in far too many places.

But none of the changes in society or the technology of medical care since Jesus' time can alter the call Jesus and the sick themselves continue to press upon us so insistently. Our call, as Pope John Paul II so precisely put it, is to "humanize sickness to heal the sick as a creature of God, as a brother in Christ."[3] This we can do only if we become agents of God's mercy and compassion. We must make our compassion effective in our action. We must, in the ministry of healing as in everything else, "permeate and improve the whole society."[4]

CHRISTIAN COMPASSION

Compassion is the concrete evidence that the virtue of charity is at work in the healer. It is the leitmotif of Christ's own healing. We need to understand that his compassion is more than pity or sympathy. It transcends social work, philanthropy, and government programs. It is the capacity to feel, and suffer with, the sick person. One experiences something of the predicament of illness, its fears, anxieties, temptations, its assault on the whole person, the loss of freedom and dignity, the utter vulnerability, and the alienation every illness produces or portends. The healer suffers something of the patient's suffering. But true compassion is more than feeling. It flows over into a willingness, desire, and intent to help, to make some sacrifice, to go out of one's way, as the Good Samaritan did. "No one can help anyone without entering with his whole person into the painful situation; without taking the risk of becoming hurt, wounded, or even destroyed in the process."[5] This love is a love that might break the health care professional. As such, it moves far beyond mere "provision" of care.[6]

The Christian must recognize with the utmost humility that compassion is a human quality shared by many outside the Christian community. We need only recall how the Stoic physicians of old had already spoken of the sick person as a brother or sister deserving of loving care.[7] What is different for the Christian is that compassion is an "obedient response to a loving Father," not "a noble act of self sacrifice,"[8] an act of humility, not of hubris. Compassion entails a comprehension of the suffering experienced by another. When we have suffered ourselves we are sometimes better able to understand it in others. As Miguel de Unamuno says, "Suffering is the substance of life and the root of personality, for only suffering makes us persons";[9] or as the Italian proverb puts it, "Illness tells us who we are."

Compassion for the suffering of others thus enriches our own understanding of what we, too, must some day pass through. It teaches us that "merciful love is never a unilateral act."[10] Compassion helps us, therefore, to realize that our sick brothers and sisters are not alien to us. They are still very much part of the human family. They are vital to our own spiritual growth. The healthy need the sick to humanize them as much as the sick need us to humanize their sickness. For it is "anguish experienced in ourselves which reveals God to us and makes us place our love in him."[11]

COMPASSION IN ACTION

Be compassionate as your Father is compassionate.[12] How does this translate into action today for the health professional, for the whole Christian community and its institutions?

For health professionals compassion is the quality that separates a mere career from a true Christian vocation. It enables us to recognize that effective as our science and technology can be, they do not remove suffering. The sick cannot escape the confrontation with mortality that even a minor illness may entail. Human illness is always illness of the whole person—body, mind, and spirit. The compassionate physician and nurse recognize that illness transcends biological aberrations in organ systems. Illness fractures our image of ourselves, upsets the balance we have struck between our aspirations and our limitations. Illness is nothing less than a forced deconstruction of the self.

Compassionate healing aims enable the healer to reconstruct the person, to help him or her to become whole again. We must heal the attack on the spirit as well as the attack on the body. The particularities of culture, ethnicity, language make illness a unique experience for each of us. True healing can only take place when all of these particulars are taken into account[13] and made part of the care that healing entails. The patient who cannot be cured by medical sciences—the chronically ill, the mentally retarded, the psychotic—may still be "healed." Even the dying patient can be healed if we help him to understand the meanings of suffering—the opening it offers to reconciliation, atonement, and sharing of Christ's suffering on the cross. This aspect of care is unique to Christian healing and notably absent in even the nobler expressions of healing outside the Christian tradition. The absence is one of the reasons it is tempting for compassion, divorced from Christian faith, to resort to assisted suicide and active, voluntary, involuntary, and nonvoluntary euthanasia. Assisted suicide and euthanasia were practices common among pagan peoples.

CHRISTIAN COMPASSION AND MEDICAL ETHICS

A commitment to Christian compassion shapes and focuses the way we interpret and apply the three major principles that dominate medical ethics today—beneficence, justice, and autonomy. It makes all of medical ethics subservient to charity, the ordering virtue.[14]

Beneficence must go well beyond the minimalistic interpretation of avoiding harm. It must entail helping others even when that involves inconvenience, sacrifice, and a degree of risk to our own self-interest. This construal of beneficence is at risk when altruism and self-interest are in conflict, as they are today. We see that conflict in many physicians' activities, e.g., in refusing to treat AIDS patients for fear of infection, in withdrawing from or withholding obstetrical and neurosurgical care for fear of malpractice, or in acting as medical entrepreneurs or gatekeepers or striking for higher pay. These practices deny the primacy of caring for the patient, which is at the heart of any charity-based medical ethic. Effacement of self-interest in the interests of the virtue of charity is crucial if we really treat the sick as our brothers and sisters.

The principle of justice is, likewise, transformed. It becomes charitable justice—not a strict blindfolded weighing of what is owed on the scales. Charitable justice is modulated by mercy—that is to say, it affords some degree of leniency where strict accounting would be expected or deserved. Charitable justice removes the blindfold, opens its eyes to the predicament of the person, and reshapes what is "just" in the light of what is seen. As Pope John Paul II has pointed out, "True mercy is, so to speak, the most profound source of justice."[15] Thus, Christian justice is charitable justice with its roots in God's love for all persons and its fulfillment in the paschal mystery.[16] On this view, all humans have just claims on those things their fellows and society can provide that ensure the dignity of the person and the value of each human life.

Finally, Christian compassion comprehends and respects the moral claim of autonomy. Autonomy becomes more than a negative principle asserted against the physician to avoid unwanted care. Charity gives autonomy a positive content as well. It recognizes the dignity of the sick as full participants in their own healing. We violate the humanity of the sick when, even in the name of benevolence, we ignore their decisions and their spiritual or personal values. This is the very antithesis of the humanization of illness compassion seeks and of the Christian concern for enabling each person to act in accordance with his or her conscience. It requires a positive effort to make a patient's moral choices as authentic as the situation permits.

When charity is the ordering virtue, it raises healing care to an act of grace, and the profession of medicine to a Christian vocation. Even practices that are not positively immoral become unacceptable, e.g., excessive vigor in collecting even just fees, impatience and insensitivity with difficult patients, or failing to be available and accessible. To treat the sick as brothers and sisters calls for a level of dedication above the ordinary.

Charitable compassion leaves no room for pejorative judgments about who is worthy or deserving of the professional's attention. There can be no place for the attitudes of some physicians (young and old) who cut corners with, or refuse treatment to, unsavory characters, e.g., drug addicts, alcoholics, or rude, dirty, or self-abusing patients. The Christian physician is not the judge of others' behavior or accountability. He or she is there to help, heal, and care for even the unlovable. This is what charity means.

Still, all who care for the sick must remember that well people are also our brothers and sisters, equally deserving our solicitude. We must balance our obligations to family, self, and community as well as to the sick. There is no universal formula to tell each of us where to strike that balance. Charity must be our guide here, too.

COMPASSION AND THE HEALING COMMUNITY

The responsibility for healing is not to be totally delegated to professionals or to social or governmental agencies. It must be shared by every member and every level of a Christian community.

The family remains the basic unit of Christian healing. Here those intimate dimensions of faith and love are to be found that are impossible to attain with strangers or institutions. Here mutual stewardship for loving care is best expressed. Here the agonizing decisions about costs, discontinuance of life support measures, or institutionalization of the aged must be made with compassion. Here, too, the sick can be supported by personal and community prayer, celebration of the Eucharist (which is a sacrament of unity), and anointing of the sick (the sacrament of hope). Here, too, Job's puzzlement—"Why, O Lord, why? Why me?"—will most insistently be asked. It is in the supportive milieu of the family that this often will be answered and shared suffering can lead to spiritual growth of all who care for the dying.

But the family should not be alone. The healing resources of the parish must be there also to relieve, strengthen, and help through visits to the sick by friends and the clergy, and by offering volunteer services, financial assistance, help in homemaking, etc.

Finally, family and parish are embedded in the larger community. If it is to be truly Christian, the whole community must make a collective commitment to charitable justice, to caring and being present to the sick.[17] A caring society will assure that the care of the sick, which is among the more rudimentary goods for a fully human life, is distributed equitably. A Christian and compassionate society cannot relegate healing to the caprices of the marketplace, competition, or medical entrepreneurs. It must see to it that the requisite social institutions and mechanisms are in place to ensure a compassionate distribution of resources for care of the sick. In the Christian healing community, medical knowledge is not proprietary. It is held in trust by professionals and society. The whole community will be disposed to make the fiscal sacrifices involved in decisions to allocate resources according to the demands of compassion and not primarily fiscal exigency.

Illness is itself disruptive of the community. God is the healer not just of individuals but of the whole community. The whole community in turn must participate in its own healing. It is God's love for the people of God that is the ultimate taproot for the compassion we are called upon to show for our sick brothers and sisters. Yet there remains much we still must do if we are to ensure that the health care ministry is to remain "one of the most vital apostolates of the ecclesial community and one of the most significant services which Christianity offers to society in the name of Jesus Christ."[18]

In the years ahead more of the responsibility must fall almost entirely on the shoulders of the laity.[19] Personal and financial sacrifices will be required to fill in the gaps left by philanthropy and government. The whole community, Christian and non-Christian, must ensure that fiscal exigency will not drive Catholic hospitals into either moral compromise or bankruptcy. No matter what health care reform looks like, it will not meet all needs, present promises to the contrary. No bureaucratic plan can ever substitute for the compassionate care and healing truly Christian health professionals and institutions must provide. If such a plan substitutes for the kind of compassionate healing we have been discussing, then it borders on hypocrisy.

When we are in doubt or falter—for the task is formidable—we can turn to the Holy Father's inspiring words on human suffering. And we can also thank him for encouraging the entire Christian community in its efforts to be a true healing community.

THE RELATION OF CARING AND CURING

What is the relationship between caring and curing? What are the moral obligations of healers—physicians, nurses, all who come into direct, hands-on contact with sick people?

It is interesting to note the differences in the ways the words "cure" and "care" are constructed in Latin and English.[20] In Latin, the noun cure comes from *cura, curae;* the verb cure comes from *curo, curare, curavi, curatum.* Both words mean essentially the same thing—to take care of, to take trouble, to be solicitous, to treat medically and surgically, to heal, to restore to health. In their English usage, cure also comes from the Latin, but care comes from Teutonic and Old English roots: to care means to be sorrowful, grieved, to lament, but also to be concerned, to feel interest, to care for, and to take care of.

In this work, we would hold that cure in the radical sense can occur without caring. Of course, a truly radical cure (*vide infra*) is one good way to care for a patient, but it is not the same as healing. Healing is a more comprehensive term than curing. It implies making the patient whole again. Even if a disease is cured, the patient may not be entirely healed. For healing to occur, the physician or nurse must also care for the patient, that is to say, be sufficiently concerned to attend to restoring health psychosocially as well as to eradicating identifiable disease.

The word "cure" now often is used in a radical sense—to refer to the eradication of the cause of an illness or disease, to the radical interruption and reversal of the natural history of the disorder. On this view a cure restores a patient at least to the state of functioning he or she enjoyed before the onset of the illness and possibly to even a better state. The possibility of cure in this sense turns on the availability of scientific medicine and radically effective therapeutic modalities, which make it possible to cure without caring.

Specific, radical, and effective cures, in the technical sense, have become available in the greatest profusion during the lifetime of physicians who entered the profession following World War II. Before that time, largely through empirical good fortune, some truly effective cures existed (cinchona bark for malaria, foxglove for heart failure, mercury for syphilis), and some were discovered by scientific investigation earlier in this century (insulin, liver extract, sulfonamides). But the golden era of specific therapy has just begun and its future promises are still to be fully apprehended.[21] We are now in the era of designer drugs, natural and man-made agents designed to attack the molecular and cellular sources of disease. Surgeons can invade any body cavity to excise, reconstruct, or replace by transplant diseased organs and tissues. Radical cure and restoration—not simply amelioration or disease containment—have become realistic and legitimate goals of medicine.

It is easy, and perhaps some think it desirable, to forget that the greater part of the history of medicine was based on a different meaning of "cure"—that associated with *care* of the ill and sick. To be sure, the extensive pharmacopoeias of the Chinese, Indian, and Roman physicians resulted from the search for curative powers. Some items in them, fortuitously, did cure; most were worthless, or even decidedly dangerous. Cure, if it did occur, resulted largely from the body's self-healing powers, and the physician's compassion, caring, encouragement, and emotional support.

The ancient grounding of medicine in care and compassion is seriously challenged by the biomedical model that defines medicine simply as applied biology.[22] On this approach, the primary function of medicine is to cure, and this requires that the physician be primarily a scientist. This model still includes containment of illness by slowing down its progress and by amelioration of its symptoms. But it focuses on *things* to do for a particular disease that are measurably effective, not the personal involvement of the health care professional in the suffering life of the sick person.

CARING AND COMPASSION?

Let us now examine what we mean by caring and how a clear concept of its full meaning is necessary to understand the religious foundation of health care and the reformulation of professional ethics. Our comments apply to all health professionals, not just to physicians. All are joined in a common task of healing, helping, and caring, and in these endeavors, the same moral obligations bind all of them similarly.

Patricia Benner and Judith Wrubel suggest that caring is a "way of being in the world."[23] They mean that caring attends to a person's sense of being taken care of therapeutically. By such therapy individual patients are assured that their experience of stress with disease (being ill) is all right. But this is not enough. The professional cares therapeutically by identifying available coping options. The professional, therefore, enters into the patient's suffering and helps reconstruct life plans based on values.[24] Thus, caring is a moral art, primary for any health care practice.

Erich Loewy suggests that caring is a biological phenomenon rooted in our emotions and feelings of compassion inseparable from, but not reducible to, the biological substrate of sentient life. While Rousseau talks about even primitive man being endowed with an innate sense of pity, Loewy expands this notion to argue that biologically based compassion is the root of the moral impulse itself.[25] This conception appears too limited; it gives to compassion a certain determinist bent that is belied by the enormous range of possible responses humans exhibit to suffering—from the sacrificial love of Mother Teresa to the sadism of Nazi physicians. In our view, caring is a much more complex phenomenon, however biological its roots might be.

There are at least four senses in which the word "care" can be understood in the health professions.

1) Compassion

The first sense is care as compassion—being concerned for another person, feeling, sharing something of his or her experience of illness and pain, being touched by the plight of another person. To care in this sense is to see the person who is ill and at the center of our ministrations as more than the object of our ministrations—as a fellow human whose experiences we cannot penetrate fully but can be touched by because we share the same humanity. Being touched can only occur if health professionals are open to their own humanity and to its implications in the healing encounter. This can often be the greatest challenge to health professionals.

2) Assistance in Living

The second sense of caring is to do for another what he or she cannot do for himself or herself. This entails assisting with all the activity of daily living compromised by illness—feeding, bathing, clothing, meeting personal needs, physical, social, and emotional. Physicians do little or none of this kind of care. Nurses do much more but less than they used to do. A large part of this care is given by nurse's aides in today's team nursing. Yet for most people, loss of the activities of daily living is the biggest rupture caused by illness in their lives. Restoring the capacity to engage in those activities and assisting people to perform them again are major elements of curing.

3) Assurance

The third sense of caring is to take care of the problem, to invite the patient to transfer to the physician or nurse responsibility and anxiety about what is wrong and what can and should be done. This is the assurance that all appropriate knowledge, skill, and personnel will be directed to the problem the patient presents, and thereby altering favorably the natural history of the disease. Assurance includes, but is not limited to, the healing power of the healing professional as a person.

4) Competence

The fourth sense of caring is to "take care," i.e., to carry out all the necessary procedures—personal and technical—with conscientious attention to detail and with perfection. This is a corollary of the third sense of caring but it places its emphasis on the craftsmanship of medicine. Together the third and fourth senses are what most health professionals would subsume under the rubric of "competence."

These four senses of care are not really separable in the optimal clinical practice. Nonetheless, in reality they are often separated, and even placed in opposition with each other. Or only one is adopted, to the exclusion of the others. For example, the biomedical model of the physician-patient relationship places emphasis on technical competence and conscientiousness, relegating the first two senses—which are more affective than technical—to other health professionals. On the other hand, the expansionist models of medicine—such as the holistic or biopsychosocial—embrace all dimensions of care, blurring the distinctions between them. Partitioning or conflating of the four senses of care leads to either neglect of one aspect or presumption of too much under the rubric of one of them. Both are perilous to the patient.

It is essential that each sense of caring be recognized for its contribution to the healing relationship. Each must be placed in its proper place in an order of priorities determined by the needs of the particular patient. While it has four dimensions, ultimately care is of one piece. The challenge to health professionals is to attend to each sense of care and to relate one to the other so that they enhance the healing relationship for each patient.

In the ideal healing relationship of patient-physician or patient-nurse, each health professional would attend to each dimension of care in every ministration. When this is not possible—as in contemporary care—these four senses of care must be at least provided by some conscious partitioning of functions among members of the medical or health care team. The moment we make such divisions, we must appreciate that the unity of care is threatened. Special attention must then be given to see that no dimension of care is neglected because none of the health care team members accepts the responsibility or sees it as proper to his or her professional tasks or status.[26]

Integral care, that is to say, care that satisfies the four senses we have defined, is a moral obligation of health professionals. It is not an option they can exercise and interpret in terms of some idiosyncratic definition of professional responsibility. The moral obligation arises out of the special human relationship that binds one who is ill to one who offers to help.

When that relationship is interpreted in terms of Christian charity, patients are brothers and sisters in the family of persons, created by God. Responsiveness to all the dimensions of caring is essential if the Christian physician or nurse is to be authentically Christian. Without denying the biological or phenomenal roots of care suggested by Loewy, Benner, and Wrubel, Christian belief cannot rest in these naturalistic explanations alone. Compassion, caring, and charitable feelings toward others are built into human nature by God and come ultimately from him, as does all that is good in us. By caring for the sick, in all the richness of that term, we are fulfilling a disposition to the good that God has implanted in us by nature. The varying degree of care exhibited by humans is an expression of the degree to which we have accepted or rejected the grace God gives us to behave compassionately toward all of our fellow persons in the human community.

CONCLUSION

Compassion in the full and authentic Christian sense is inspired in us because in every suffering human we recognize Christ, who suffered for all of us. The Crucifixion is repeated daily in every mortally sick person. We know that without it there can be no Easter Sunday. We know, too, that caring extends to the very moment of abandonment, when the sick person places his soul and body in the care of God, trusts in that caring, and through that caring enters into the only thing that will heal completely, union with a caring God. Here we are beyond biology, psychology, and philosophy, which can at best intimate the sources of caring, but only faintly and vaguely.

NOTES

1. St. Thomas Aquinas, *Summa Theologiae* [Vol. 34], trans. and ed. R. J. Batten (New York: Blackfriars, 1975), II-II, q. 31, a. 4, pp. 232–235.

2. Mark 1:32–34, in *The New American Bible* (New York: Catholic Book Publishing, 1970), p. 44.

3. Pope John Paul II, "Humanize Hospital Work [Address to the Sixty-First General Chapter of the Hospital Order of St. John of God]," *L'Osservatore Romano* 16, no. 4 (No. 768) (January 24, 1983): 3.

4. "Decree on the Apostolate of the Laity," in *The Documents of Vatican II*, ed. Walter M. Abbott (New York: Crossroad, 1989), pp. 489–521.

5. Henri Nouwen, *The Wounded Healer* (New York: Doubleday, 1972), p. 72.

6. Jean Vanier, *The Broken Body: Journey to Wholeness* (London: Darton, Longman and Todd, 1988); Kathryn Spink, *Jean Vanier and L'Arche: A Communion of Love* (New York: Crossroad, 1991). L'Arche communities in twenty-two nations attempt to demonstrate the Gospel imperative.

7. Owsei Temkin and Lillian Temkin, eds., *Ancient Medicine: Selected Papers of Ludwig Edelstein* (Baltimore: Johns Hopkins Press, 1967), pp. 345 and 337–340.

8. Donald P. McNeill, Douglas A. Morrison, and Henri Nouwen, eds., *Compassion: A Reflection on the Christian Life* (New York: Doubleday, 1982), p. 42.

9. Miguel de Unamuno, *The Tragic Sense of Life*, trans. A. Kerrigan (Princeton: Bollingen Series, 1972), p. 224.

10. Pope John Paul II, *Encyclical Letter: Dives in Misericordia* (Washington: U.S. Catholic Conference, 1981), p. 45.

11. Unamuno, *Tragic Sense*, p. 227.

12. Luke 6:36, in *The New American Bible* (New York: Catholic Book Publishing, 1970), 76.

13. Edmund D. Pellegrino and David C. Thomasma, *Helping and Healing* (Washington: Georgetown University Press, 1996).

14. Edmund D. Pellegrino, "Agape and Ethics: Some Reflections of Medical Morals from a Catholic Christian Perspective," in *Catholic Perspectives in Medical Morals*, ed. Edmund D. Pellegrino, John P. Langan, and John C. Harvey (Dordrecht, Netherlands and Boston: Kluwer, 1989), pp. 277–300.

15. Pope John Paul II, *Dives in Misericordia*, p. 46.

16. David Hollenbach, "Modern Catholic Teachings Concerning Justice," in *The Faith That Does Justice*, ed. J. C. Haughey (New York: Paulist Press, 1977), p. 226.

17. Pope Paul VI, *The Encyclical Letter on the Development of Peoples* (Washington: U.S. Catholic Conference, 1967).

18. Pope John Paul II, "Address to the Catholic Health Association," *L'Osservatore Romano* (September 21, 1987): 19.

19. Kevin D. O'Rourke, *Reasons for Hope: Laity in Catholic Health Care Facilities* (St. Louis: Catholic Health Association of the United States, 1983).

20. *"Cura,"* in *Oxford Latin Dictionary* (Oxford: Clarendon Press, 1983), pp. 473–474. *"Curo,"* in *Oxford Latin Dictionary* (Oxford: Clarendon Press, 1983), pp. 475–476. *"Cure,"* in *Oxford English Dictionary* (Oxford: Clarendon Press, 1961), Vol. 2, p. 1263. *"Care,"* in *Oxford English Dictionary* (Oxford: Clarendon Press, 1961), Vol. 2, pp. 115–16.

21. Edmund D. Pellegrino, "The Sociocultural Impact of Twentieth-Century Therapeutics," in *The Therapeutic Revolution: Essays in the Social History of American Medicine*, ed. Morris J. Vogel and Charles E. Rosenberg (Philadelphia: University of Pennsylvania Press, 1979), pp. 245–266.

22. Donald Seldin, "The Medical Model: Biomedical Science as the Basis of Medicine," in *Beyond Tomorrow* (New York: Rockefeller University Press, 1977).

23. Patricia Benner and Judith Wrubel, *The Primacy of Caring* (Menlo Park, Cal.: Addison-Wesley, 1989), p. xi.

24. Edmund D. Pellegrino and David C. Thomasma, *For the Patient's Good: Toward the Restoration of Beneficence in Health Care* (New York: Oxford University Press, 1988), pp. 73–91.

25. Erich Loewy, *Suffering and the Beneficent Community* (Albany: State University of New York Press, 1991).

26. David C. Thomasma, "A Code of Ethics for Interdisciplinary Care: A Working Paper," *Proceedings of the Eighth Annual Conference on Interdisciplinary Health Team Care* (Columbus, Ohio: Ohio State University School of Allied Health Professions and Commission on Interprofessional Education and Practice, 1986), pp. 1–16.

7

Prudential Judgment and Religious Commitment

> *The religious truth is essential if we are to make sense out of the world, make an order out of it, which is not imposed for our own purposes.*
>
> — Martin C. D'Arcy, *Humanism and Christianity*.[1]

The three theological virtues are indispensable dispositions of character that, taken together, constitute that orientation of our personal lives we call a religious commitment. This assumes possession of the natural moral virtues.[2] But, as we have emphasized up to this point, the theological virtues go beyond the natural virtues, complementing and supplementing them by the imprints of faith, hope, and charity on our personal, public, and professional lives. In this chapter, we will explicate more specifically how a religious commitment makes a difference in the health professional's clinical moral judgments, the daily decisions at the bedside.

We will argue that religious belief cannot, and should not, be isolated from medical ethics, that it is an essential counterpoint to the secularism of ethical discourse today, and that serious objections to intermingling faith and reason in clinical decisions in a morally pluralistic society can be met satisfactorily. Our focus for this purpose will be on the *process* of clinical ethical decisions and not their substantive content. This is not to depreciate the substantive moral content of the acts in question—whether they be abortion, euthanasia, in vitro fertilization, or genetic screening. A morally defensible clinical decision must be right and good substantively, and it also must be made in a morally defensible way.

There are several good reasons for concentrating on the process of making moral choices in medicine. First, it is a substantive requirement of Christian morality itself to practice the natural virtues in our dealings with our fellow human beings. Even if our choices are intrinsically right and good when we make them jointly with others or when we carry them out, we must do so with charitable concern. Second, the procedural dimension has received less attention by religious ethicists, who have focused, properly enough, on the moral acts themselves. Third, there is more likelihood of agreement with secularists on procedure than on substantive normative ethics. This is an important practical issue since we live in a pluralistic society wherein, as a rule, believers and nonbelievers must make decisions together—as professionals, family, and team members. In this, we realize that procedure and substance are not neatly separable, but it is useful and important to disengage them at least for heuristic purposes.

For these reasons, Christian physicians must comprehend more clearly how important procedural ethics has become as a meeting ground in which believers and nonbelievers have a reasonable possibility and probability of agreeing. This convergence must not obscure the differences in substantive ethics. Even the way procedural ethics is pursued may be shaped by the presence or absence of religious commitment. The integration of Christian commitment into clinical decisions does not exhaust the possibilities of a Christian vocation to medicine. But it offers concrete opportunity for frequent and practical dialogue with colleagues, families, and patients who may hold other beliefs or none at all. Engaging in this dialogue as a Christian is part of the vocation of transforming the contemporary culture, of which John Paul II has spoken so often as incumbent on each of us in accord with the station in life we occupy.[3]

Three questions seem most important to the point of view we are espousing: (1) What is the justification for introducing religious belief into clinical decisions in a morally pluralistic society? (2) What specifically do such commitments contribute to decision making? (3) What is the proper relationship between faith and reason in clinical ethics?

We approach these questions from personal experience—one of us as a clinician and ethicist, the other as a clinically oriented philosopher. While we focus on medical decision making, our conclusions are applicable by analogy to other health professionals and to professionals outside the health field as well.

WHY INCLUDE RELIGIOUS COMMITMENTS IN ETHICAL DECISION MAKING?

Several objections to integrating faith commitments into clinical ethics will occur immediately to believers and nonbelievers alike. These are serious obstacles with solid foundations in history and experience. They cannot be ignored, but they can and should be overcome.

First, there is the historical evidence of conflict among Christian denominations on some of the most fundamental ethical issues. Christians start with a common belief in man's spiritual destiny, God's creative act, and the necessity of personal salvation. But some argue as utilitarians, some as deontologists, some as situation ethicists, and some as emotivists. Some believe in an unchanging, objective moral order, others in an evolving order in which man and God are cocreators. Roman Catholics draw on Sacred Scripture along with reason, tradition, and ecclesiastic authority. Other Christian denominations regard human reason as too enfeebled by Original Sin to be relied upon. Ultimately they rely on personal and prayerful interpretations of what God wants them to be and do in particular situations.

Second and equally problematic are the variations in the way Sacred Scripture is used in ethical discourse. Some take scriptural texts as literal and absolute rules. For others, Scripture offers guidelines to be followed more in the spirit than in the letter. Still others see them as enabling texts that guide the Christian in the moment of dilemma to choose rightly. Each alternative results in a different approach to ethical dilemmas, substantively as well as procedurally.

As a result, ethical discourse among Christians may end up in frustration, even on such substantive and crucial issues as abortion, euthanasia, or in vitro fertilization. Each denomination is convinced of the truth of its position and sees the others as misinterpreting the divine Commandments and God's will. In the past, conflicts of this kind within the Christian community have given rise to war, social unrest, and unedifying scandal. Worst of all, such conflicts cast doubt on the message of Christianity as a religion based in love of God and man. The religious wars and persecutions of the past are still imprinted in human memory. Even today, the uncharitable, self-righteous, and even violent attitudes of some Christians who wish to force their beliefs on others are a source of worry.

Finally, secularists argue that all persons may hold to their beliefs privately but must divorce themselves from those beliefs in public decisions or when others find them objectionable. In this view, the physician who is a Christian should keep religion and professional life in separate compartments. Secular extremists even suggest that sincere practicing Jews, Muslims, or Christians should either accept what law and/or social mores permit or disqualify themselves from practice except among those who share their beliefs. Further, while rights of conscience are avowed by many, there is a growing tendency to demand conformity to public opinion as a standard for morality, seemingly one goal of secular humanism.

In light of these objections, it may seem perverse to argue for an inclusion of religious commitment in ethical decision making. Would this not damage the emerging consensus on procedure, which has succeeded precisely because religious commitments have been excluded? Would it not undo two decades of consensus building and complicate attempts to pursue medical ethics in democratic, morally pluralistic societies? What justifications can we offer for possibly upsetting the fine balance that seems to obtain at present?

The first reason is that religious belief is an undeniable and highly significant reality in the lives of most human beings. Even in ostensibly secular societies, many still acknowledge a transcendent source of morality that demands their allegiance in moral choices. Consciously or unconsciously, these commitments shape the whole process of ethical decision making. They are the moral presuppositions upon which moral choices are ultimately made. It is in relation to them that the most serious disagreements may arise since such presuppositions are so strongly held and are so close to our personal identity. Also, they must take precedence over other considerations.

In addition, failure to account for substantive religious commitments is a tacit endorsement of procedure and analysis over substantive and normative ethics. There is much to be said for the procedural emphasis and analytical rigor of contemporary medical ethics. Nothing in this essay is meant to demean this rigor. But procedural rigor is not enough. After an ethically valid procedure has been followed, the question remains: is the resulting decision morally right and good? For the Christian physician, the ethical decision must be congruent not just with procedure but with religious commitments. The Christian physician cannot cooperate in a decision that is morally offensive, no matter how defensible the process by which it is made. *What* is decided is as morally relevant as *how* it is decided.

A competent patient may, for example, request direct assistance in suicide or voluntary euthanasia. Looked at simply from the point of view of the decision-making process, we should respect the patient's right to self-determination. But the action requested is morally unacceptable. For a Catholic Christian, if assisted suicide and even euthanasia become legal, as it very likely will in states other than Oregon where it was recently legalized by public referendum, the conflict between secular and religious norms will become as acute as it is now on the subject of abortion. Under these circumstances, the Catholic physician would be obliged to withdraw from care of the patient even though the decision was made by a competent patient in accordance with the moral and legal standards of informed consent. Clearly, the physician is as much a moral agent as the patient. Therefore, neither patient nor physician can impose values upon the other. It is important to underscore this point, since patient autonomy is virtually an absolute and overriding principle in the minds of many.

This is not to deny that the physician has an obligation to act for the good of the patient, which includes attending to all of the patient's interests—spiritual as well as medical and material.[4] To violate beliefs intrinsic to a patient's self-identity, whether religious or not, is to violate the humanity of the patient. It is an essential obligation of the healing relationship that both physician and patient recognize and respect each other's religious and other values. There are limits to how far the autonomy of one or the other may be respected if the decision-making process is to be morally equitable.

When the health professional knows or shares the patient's beliefs, he or she has a serious obligation to assist the patient to make a morally authentic decision. The professional should help the patient identify the moral issues and should suggest appropriate pastoral counseling when the patient is in spiritual doubt. Moreover, the physician ought to help the patient draw upon whatever spiritual resources the patient possesses. They often are the only effective resources for coping with the tragic choices so common in chronically debilitating or fatal diseases. This obligation is too often neglected even by Christian physicians and nurses. Praying with the patient, participating in the sacrament of anointing of the sick with patient and family, and working closely with pastoral counselors are acts of healing and charity with great meaning for the patient.

Even when the health professional is intellectually and emotionally opposed to the patient's beliefs, there is still an obligation to recognize religious values and to assist the patient to draw upon them. The physician who cannot, in good conscience, help the patient in this way to make the best possible decision should withdraw from giving care. This must always be done respectfully and without vindictiveness or rancor. To continue as the patient's physician under these circumstances is to betray the trust essential to the healing relationship. To override the patient's beliefs by deception, to ridicule them as "irrational," or to attribute them to some mental aberration is indefensible. Respect for the person's autonomy means precisely that—respect for the patient as he or she is, not as the physician wants him or her to be.

Parenthetically, it is equally indefensible to take advantage of the patient's vulnerability or anxiety for purposes of proselytization. Some Christians believe that if the patient is a nonbeliever or a fallen believer, they have an obligation to evangelize or convert by any means short of violence. It is one thing to assist the patient to find meaning or succor and to give witness to Gospel truths in one's own behavior. It is quite a different thing to force one's own beliefs upon the patient. Any "conversion" under such circumstances is morally and spiritually fraudulent. There is no need for the physician, however, to hide his or her own religious beliefs and humility in the face of an illness that no longer yields to medical ministration.

Finally, there is an obligation to take religious commitment into account in the practice of holistic medicine. Unfortunately, many who most vigorously champion the inclusion of psychosocial dimensions in holistic care of patients exclude the religious dimension. This is a peculiarly incomplete form of holism since it is virtually impossible to separate the spiritual from the personal and psychosocial elements in a patient's life. If the human person is a unity and if the full dimensions of personhood are to be respected, then the spiritual dimension cannot be ignored even by the nonbelieving physician. Healing, which means "making whole again," often requires repairing the self-identity fractured by illness. This will mean helping the patient to cope in his or her own way spiritually in confronting personal finitude, a confrontation that any serious illness presents. Taking account of religious commitments, therefore, is as essential as technical competence in achieving the end of medicine—a right and good healing action for a particular person.[5] Indeed, it is part of the definition of competent care.

HOW DOES RELIGIOUS COMMITMENT SHAPE MORAL CHOICE?

The process of moral choice in medicine is built on a four-level framework. How the participants interpret each level shapes not only the process but also the content of their moral decisions. The four levels of ethical decision making are these: (1) the conception we hold of the physician-patient relationship; (2) the way we interpret the prima facie principles of medical ethics; (3) the ethical theory we use to define the good; and (4) the ultimate sources on which we ground our whole morality. The first three levels are, in the final analysis, derived from, and shaped by, the fourth level—the ultimate source of our morality, regardless of whether one has a religious commitment.

On the first level are the conception we hold of the physician-patient interaction and the conception of healing that flows from it. A variety of models of this relationship are current today. On one view, the relationship is seen as analogous to a legal contract for services.[6] On another, it is likened to a commodity transaction similar to other commercial transactions.[7] A third view regards the healing relationship as essentially applied biology.[8] A fourth view interprets the relationship as a covenant of trust in which the physician is expected to act primarily in the best interests of the patient even if that requires effacement of his own personal interests.[9] Obviously, the ethics of the relationship will vary with the model we accept. If the relationship is a contract, the ethics of law prevails; if it is applied biology, the ethics of science; if it is a business transaction, the ethics of the market place; and if it is a covenant, the ethics of virtue and trust.

The second level in the decision-making structure is the way we construe the three prima facie principles of medical ethics—beneficence, autonomy, and justice—and their three derivative duties—truth telling, promise keeping, and confidentiality. Each principle is open to a variety of interpretations.

Beneficence, for example, may be limited to simple nonmaleficence. It may be taken as doing good for the patient as long as it means no inconvenience for the doctor. On a higher level, it might entail a positive duty to act in the patient's interest even at the cost of financial loss or physical risk for the doctor. At the highest level, beneficence might entail, as with Mother Teresa, heroic self-sacrifice in the interests of the sick and the poor.

Autonomy may, in like fashion, be interpreted variously. For some, respect for autonomy might mean absolute subservience to the patient's will regardless of what the patient requests. Others might place limits on autonomy when the patient requests something that either violates the physician's moral values, harms someone else, or results in harm to the patient him- or herself. Since the locus of decision making has shifted from the doctor to the patient in the last twenty years, the precise construal we place on autonomy markedly influences the process of moral choice.

The principle of justice has many interpretations as well. Is it to be defined on the basis of equity, merit, social position, power, need, or ability to pay? Does society owe any special obligation to the sick person? How we distribute any scarce health care resource will be determined directly by what meaning we attribute to justice.

At the third level in medical-ethical decision making is the choice of an ethical theory, e.g., deontology, consequentialism, subjectivism, virtue, etc. Each theory is based in some conception of the good. Is that good to be utility, adherence to duty, the categorical imperative, self-interest, human nature, divine revelation, or spiritual destiny? Each conception of the good will provide different answers to the concrete ethical dilemmas encountered in clinical practice. This is particularly true when the subjects of our concern are the vulnerable, the poor, the aged, or infants, all of whose social utility is compromised and who, as a consequence, are thrown upon society's mercy.

The positions we take at these first three levels of decision making (the levels of the physician-patient relationship, of ethical principles, and of ethical theory) cannot be divorced from the commitments we make at the fourth and most fundamental level—the level of the foundational sources of our morality. At this level, every human being makes a commitment to some view of the world, man, and the existence or nonexistence of a transcendent order. This fourth level forms the irreducible source of a person's morality, the final justification for what he or she thinks is right and good.

For some, the individual is the creator of his own values and the sole determinant of what is right and good. For others, the ultimate source of morality is the appeal to unaided human reason, i.e., to philosophical ethics. Many others would make the texts of Sacred Scripture the sole arbiter of moral good. These are the fundamentalists and fideists, who seek specific and concrete moral prescriptions from the Bible and reject rational argumentation as irrelevant. Another view is that of the Roman Catholic moral tradition, in which reason and revelation, as well as ecclesiastical authority, are accepted sources of morality, each offering its own unique contribution. At the opposite pole are those for whom biology or sociobiology are the ultimate sources of morality. For them, the preservation of the species is the ultimate good for individuals and society. Finally, an increasing segment of the population roots its morality in culture and history, claiming preference for an ever-changing morality with no fixed principles except the principle of change, in a societal context where standards of moral accountability in the external community have eroded.

Clearly the moral positions we take depend on which of these ultimate sources of morality we accept. This can best be illustrated by showing how a commitment to Catholic Christianity might alter the choices we would make at each of the four levels in the process of ethical decision making.

First, a commitment to Roman Catholic Christianity provides a philosophical anthropology upon which to base the three ethical principles used in medical-moral decisions. The lack of such an agreed-upon anthropology in contemporary ethics is a major reason for many of its frustrations. The principles of beneficence, autonomy, and justice, for example, are taken by contemporary ethical theory to be prima facie principles. But they lack grounding in something more fundamental, such as a theory of human nature. Without such a theory, it is difficult to validate these prima facie principles, and they become self-justifying "absolutes."

This is not the place to elaborate on or defend the Christocentric anthropology of Roman Catholicism. It is important, however, to show how this philosophy of man shapes ethical choice. Humans, in the Roman Catholic view, are creatures of God, composites of body and spirit oriented to a spiritual destiny and called to personal salvation and to a concern for the salvation of other men and women. This is the conception of Christian humanism that Pope John Paul II saw as sufficiently important to make the topic of his first encyclical, *Redemptor Hominis.*[10] This view of man gives a meaning to human existence beyond immediate human intentions, desires, and needs. It ascribes an intrinsic value to each human life. It grounds so-called prima facie principles such as respect for persons, beneficence, and justice in the obligations owed to humans as humans, as creatures of God. It incorporates the "comprehensiveness of the Christian philosophy," the heavenly promises, and the cross "embodied in its creed."[11]

On this view of the dignity of human nature, certain decisions (such as abortion or euthanasia) are never permissible. Consequentialism, moral subjectivism, and relativism would be inadmissible as primary ethical theories. Also, the physician-patient relationship could never be treated as a commercial contract, as an exercise in applied biology, or as the repair of body parts. Beneficence would be more than mere nonmaleficence. Autonomy would never be absolute, nor would justice be based on the ability to pay.

A second way this religious perspective alters ethical decisions is by giving meaning to illness and death. For Christians, suffering and death are not the unmitigated evils they are to the contemporary world. Viewed from the perspective of Christian theology, every suffering human life takes on meaning.[12] Illness becomes an enabling, rather than a uniformly disabling, experience. It can serve various purposes such as reconciliation with God, atonement for past sins, a source of example and inspiration to others. It can draw families to greater love for each other in their solicitude for a sick or dying member.

Christians recognize that suffering is the way of the cross that Christ chose to journey and that he foretold each of us must journey. The Christocentric view of human nature also answers Job's dilemma. Why must the just man suffer? For Job, the answer came in face-to-face confrontation with God's majesty as Creator of a world whose purposes Job would never be able to fully fathom. For the Christian, identification with Christ's suffering gives a meaning to human suffering that requires no logical exposition or defense of the kind Job and his friends sought from the Lord. Job finally ended by surrendering to the majesty of God without knowing God's reasons. The Christian surrenders because he has an ineffable model in Christ, whom he is called to emulate.

On this view of suffering, utilitarian or sympathetic impulses to shorten human life deliberately, to devalue the "quality" or economic worth of the lives of disabled infants, the aged, the retarded, or the handicapped would be morally indefensible. Quality of life, economics, or social worth could not be defended as criteria for withholding or withdrawing life-sustaining treatment in comatose patients. For the Christian, each human life has meaning, given it by God and not by men. Even if we cannot divine that meaning, we must recognize it in every life we encounter.

A naturalistic ethic, without a grounding in religious commitments, leaves a gap between cognition of the right and good and the motivation to *do* the right and to be good. This is singled out as one of the major problems in contemporary moral philosophy, which hopes that a better understanding of moral psychology will close this gap.[13] As a result, some moral theorists turn to psychology to "purify" our motives of aberrant psychological drives in order to move us more surely from knowing to doing the good.[14]

Without depreciating these efforts to understand our moral motivations, it does not seem likely that the gap between cognition and motivation can be closed by more cognition. On the other hand, a genuine commitment to a Christian way of life closes that gap immediately. For the Christian, to recognize what is right and good is to be motivated to do it. Obviously, in actual practice, many Christians recognize the good yet avoid or suppress it and do evil. When this occurs, they recognize that they have fallen from or rejected God's grace. This is very different from recognizing the good and not acknowledging any obligation to do it.

For the Christian, to act morally is a command from God defined in scriptural texts such as the Decalogue or the Sermon on the Mount. The Decalogue is precise in its admonitions, the Gospel less so but equally compelling. The enlightened Christian seeks to act out of love, not out of fear. Failing this, however, God's call to do his will, to live in accord with his commandments, and to love one's neighbor is unequivocal.

Christian commitment, in addition, provides an ordering principle that can resolve conflicts between moral principles. This is the ordering principle of charity, the supernatural virtue that calls for genuinely unselfish acts on behalf of our fellow men and women. Charity is the summation of Christ's own mission, which Christians are called upon to emulate. Charity is a virtue that transforms each prima facie moral principle and raises it to the level of grace. Charitable beneficence entails a clear effacement of self-interest in the interests of the sick person; charitable justice goes beyond what is strictly owed to embrace preferentially those who are poor or rejected or especially vulnerable; charitable respect for persons is more than a legalistic recognition of the rights to autonomy and privacy.

Charity does not ignore ethical principle or substitute vague moral sentiment for rational ethical decisions. It does, however, ask how each principle applies in the light of the Sermon on the Mount or the example of Jesus' daily healing work. It emphasizes the kind of persons we ought to be rather than the particular solution to a moral puzzle. Charity thus restores virtue to a central place in moral philosophy. In this sense, it coincides with philosophical ethics' most recent trend, which attempts to restore character and virtue to moral behavior.[15]

This emphasis on virtue—whether natural or supernatural—is particularly significant for biomedical ethics. It is the very theme of this book. A patient, given the predicament of illness, is vulnerable, dependent, and compelled to trust the physician. Every action decided upon finally must be channeled through the physician, who carries out the decision whether it is made by a competent patient, the surrogate of an incompetent patient, or a legal guardian. In every medical act, it is the physician who must interpret the spirit of the patient's wishes and interests. The physician's character stands inevitably between the patient and harm. No contract for service, no informed consent, no hospital or public policy can anticipate the exigencies of every therapeutic moment. One might argue justifiably for limitations on the physician's discretionary latitude, but not all trust can be eliminated. The virtue of fidelity to the patient's interests and to the promise of beneficence implicit in the healing relationship is central to the physician's morality. It is the final safeguard against those subtle temptations to use the patient's exploitable predicament to self-advantage.

A Christian perspective not only puts the focus on virtue; it defines charity as the ordering virtue. The classical cardinal virtues—prudence, temperance, fortitude, and justice—are not ignored. Rather, they are nuanced, ordered, and elevated in sensitivity by charity, as is the whole analytical process requisite for rational decision making.

A Christian perspective also buffers the strong individualistic trend of so much of contemporary biomedical ethics.[16] Christianity is community-centered. It eschews the moral atomism of the libertarian or the absolutist interpretation of the principle of autonomy. Patient and physician are united with each other and the larger community. They are bonded to each other and to the larger community of others in need. They are called to foster each other's welfare and to do so as children of a common Father. The sick remain members of the Christian community with a special claim on the community's solicitude.

Finally, the Christian physician practices his or her profession not as a mere occupation or career but as a vocation. The Christian shares with all men and women the obligation to respond to God's double call—to personal salvation and to help in the salvation of those with whom we come into daily contact. The peculiar nature of medicine as a human activity makes a vocation to medicine a vehicle with special salvific opportunities. As Thomas Merton puts it: "The differences between the various vocations lie in the different ways each enables man to discover God's love, appreciate it, respond to it, and share it with others. Each vocation has for its aim the propagation of the divine life in the world."[17]

The physician who seeks to practice the profession as a true Christian vocation knows its spiritual possibilities cannot be exhausted, and has always presented the image of Christ the Divine Healer, a model who must be emulated but can never be equaled. The Christian physician must be thoroughly competent and must, through daily work, propagate "the divine life in the world," as Thomas Merton so well put it.

A Christian vocation to medicine calls for an integration of what it is to be a physician with what it is to be a Christian. Profession and faith cannot be isolated from each other without damage to both. To unite them has always been difficult, but never more so than today. For today the Christian physician functions in a world largely secular and morally heterogeneous. The challenges of scientific positivism, commercialism, and self-interest are direct and powerful. But even more challenging are the moral quandaries inherent in the unprecedented technological capabilities of modern medicine. As a result, a Christian vocation to medicine today entails the obligation to make one's faith commitment an explicit part of ethical decision making.

As mentioned before, integrating Christian ethics into clinical decision making does not exhaust the possibilities of a Christian vocation to medicine. The substantive and normative content of religious tradition and moral theology must be integrated as well. And both must be accompanied by dedicated service to the sick in charity, patience, and courage.

THE RELATIONSHIP OF FAITH AND REASON IN MEDICAL DECISIONS

At the outset, we listed some substantial objections to taking religious commitment into account in ethical decision making. These objections are not trivial, and they must always be kept in mind if the current dialogue in medical ethics is not to degenerate into unproductive and recriminatory debates that undermine the growing consensus on procedural ethics. To avoid this, the responsibility is heavy on the committed Christian to engage in ethical dialogue without sacrificing either analytical rigor or the integrity of his or her faith. Parochial assertions without rational argument, on the one hand, and facile compromise of principle simply for the sake of consensus, on the other, are equally self-defeating. They frustrate the effort to take religious commitment into account. They also reinforce the skeptic's suspicion that

Christian ethics ultimately must be irrational if it flees from rational discourse.

To avoid this kind of intellectual double jeopardy, the Christian physician is required to establish a proper relationship between right reason and right faith. This is a perennial problem for any religiously motivated intellectual who wishes to engage in intellectual discourse with the cultural ideas of his or her times. We will confine our examination of this relationship of faith and reason to the relatively narrow arena of clinical ethical decision making.

To begin with, a right relationship between faith and reason in ethical discourse requires a recognition of the epistemological distinction between these two realms, that is, between philosophical and theological ethics. Both use reason, and therefore both must follow the usual rules of logical discourse. Philosophical ethics, however, depends solely on the use of unaided human reason. Theological ethics uses the same rules of reason, but they are enriched by divine revelation. Thus, philosophical ethics accepts as evidence only what is ascertainable by reason or observation, while theological ethics begins with a faith commitment, an acceptance of the fact of revealed moral guides. In the Roman Catholic tradition, the evidence of the Scriptures is further enlarged by tradition and the teachings of the official magisterium. In theological ethics, reason is not abandoned, nor are faith and reason in contradiction. Rather, they complement and supplement each other. Much of what theological ethics posits is also derivable by reason.

In ethical dialogue with those who reject the sources of evidence that Christians admit, we must hold to these distinctions. With those who accept only philosophical argumentation, we must be willing to go as far as unaided human reason is able to go. We cannot expect to make a point simply by recitation of biblical or ecclesiastical authority. This means the discourse may go only so far. But this is not a reason for refusing to enter the discourse or breaking it off. There are several very good reasons for continuing the discussion on purely philosophical terms.

For one thing, Christians can give evidence that religious commitment is still respectful of reason—its rules as well as its limitations. Believers must be willing to expose their own positions to critical and logical scrutiny. Moreover, nonbelievers may exalt reason yet advance arguments that violate the rules of ordinary logic or are weak or incoherent. If nonbelievers are not introduced to the way those with a faith commitment justify their positions, they will never be exposed to the possibility of understanding or accepting such arguments. Finally, whether they agree or not, secular ethicists are often amazed when a believer hides or compromises his or her faith commitment.[18] Under such circumstances, it is hard to avoid the suspicion that recourse to faith is a weak, spurious, or hypocritical way of protecting a conceptually destitute position.

For these reasons, it is a moral obligation of Christians to engage in serious ethical discourse with all the participants in ethical decisions. To be sufficiently well informed and to be able to do so effectively is a requisite condition for practicing medicine as a vocation.

To be effective, a second caveat must be observed: the believer must act charitably toward what he or she may consider an erroneous or even insulting counterposition. The quickest way for a Christian to defeat this position and to discredit his or her whole faith is to act uncharitably, condescendingly, or censoriously to those with whom he or she disagrees. Such behavior undermines the claim that Christian belief can improve the moral behavior of those who profess to follow its teachings. Being charitable does not entail acceptance of a relativist ethic, as so many Catholics fear. The distinction between the beliefs a person holds and that person's status as a human being is time-honored. One can and must be respectful of others out of charity.

Another important distinction is between an immoral choice or action and personal culpability for that choice or action. No one can enter the mind of another person so completely as to weigh the competing influences of environment, internal predisposition, will, and intellect needed to judge the moral guilt of another human being. It is incongruous for Christians, who believe God is their judge, to usurp God's prerogative by pronouncing their own judgment about the guilt of others. This position is reinforced by the divine command, "Judge not that you may not be judged."

One certainly may hold to an objective order of morality and judge the objective moral validity of decisions or acts without condemning the person responsible for them. Making this distinction charitably yet unequivocally is intrinsic to the vocation of the Christian ethicist. Christian ethics is ultimately not a set of rules or a way to win ethical debates but a way of living. If charity does not form the whole human person and manifest itself in action and word, then no amount of reason will convince a nonbeliever. Correct ethical positions have been defeated too many times by the self-righteousness of the overzealous Christian. The way we engage with even the hostile opponent reveals more about the veracity of our message than our logical arguments. Every such encounter is an opportunity to give evidence that Christian ethics is a humanizing, not a dehumanizing, endeavor. To lose that opportunity is to betray the aim of Christian ethics, which is not the promulgation of abstract rules but formation of a right conscience in every human person.

Christian ethics, then, requires that we respect the persons with whom we disagree. They are to be taken seriously, listened to, and given credit for sincerely wanting to do the right and the good thing. When we disagree, we must do so without impugning motives. This does not imply acceptance of the deficiencies of a secular ethic. It does mean admitting the logical debilities of our own positions when they exist.

It is essential to admit that some of our positions as Christians are not fully defensible without recourse to those sources of evidence the secular ethicist does not accept. This accomplishes two things: first, it may help us to comprehend the degree to which we are dependent upon divine revelation, scriptural sources, or the teaching of a church, and second, it shows how a faith commitment opens alternate avenues beyond principles and logical analysis to expand the way ethical dilemmas may be examined.

In Christian ethics, as in other branches of philosophy, religious tradition owes much to the critical yet respectful way St. Thomas entered into dialogue with the pagan philosophers, learning, modifying, and expanding their thought with intelligence and charity. His is the model the Christian physician may follow with profit in the own daily dialogue with physicians, ethicists, or patients, secular or religious, when making serious moral choices.

These distinctions and correlations between reason and faith in ethics, that is, between philosophy and theology, are crucial if religious physicians are to exercise an intellectual and moral ministry as part of their healing ministry. When theology abandons or weakens its commitment to biblical revelation, ecclesiastical authority, or tradition, it becomes another philosophy among the many competing for rational acceptance. When philosophy discovers principles and concepts that expand and fulfill the higher potentialities of the human spirit, it leads to enhancing one's theology. By exhibiting both faith and reason in proper relationship with each other, the physician expands the possibilities in ethical decisions and simultaneously serves both patients and his or her faith commitment.

PERORATION

Medical ethics has expanded more rapidly in the last 20 years than in the whole of its previous 2,500-year history. That expansion has derived from a convergence of forces—the spread of democracy and public education, the rate of medical progress, the growth of moral heterogeneity, and the entry of economics, law, and politics into medical decisions.

Throughout this period, the dominant spirit of medical ethics has been philosophical, analytical, secular, and procedural. Theological ethics and religious commitment have been excluded from the general discourse. Religious conviction, however, remains a significant reality in the lives of physicians, patients, and institutions, shaping the process of ethical decision making in profound ways.

The prudent Christian physician has an obligation to take religious commitment into account in medical-ethical decisions even in a secular world. His or her education in medicine and Christian ethics makes this an intrinsic element of the medical vocation. To do so with the requisite balance of analytical rigor, fidelity to faith commitments, and charity is a service to nonbelievers as well as believers. This balance is, in any case, the special obligation of Christian professionals: "The more you know and the better you understand, the more severely will you be judged, unless your life is the more holy."[19]

In the penultimate chapter, we turn to a discussion of how the three traditional principles of bioethics are shaped differently by a Christian viewpoint. Our final chapter enunciates a Christian personalism as a synthesis of Christian virtue theory.

NOTES

1. Martin C. D'Arcy, *Humanism and Christianity* (New York: Meridian Books, 1970), p. 190.

2. Edmund D. Pellegrino and David C. Thomasma, *The Virtues in Medical Practice* (New York: Oxford University Press, 1993).

3. Pope John Paul II, *Encyclical Letter: Redemptor Hominis* (Washington: U.S. Catholic Conference, 1979); Pope John Paul II, *Encyclical Letter: Ex Corde Ecclesiae* (Washington: U.S. Catholic Conference, 1990); and Pope John Paul II, *Encyclical Letter: Veritatis Splendor* (Washington: U.S. Catholic Conference, 1994).

4. Edmund D. Pellegrino and David C. Thomasma, *For the Patient's Good: Toward the Restoration of Beneficence in Health Care* (New York: Oxford University Press, 1988).

5. Edmund D. Pellegrino, "Toward a Reconstruction of Medical Morality: The Primacy of the Act of Profession and the Fact of Illness," *Journal of Medicine and Philosophy* 4, no. 1 (1979): 32–56.

6. Robert M. Veatch, *A Theory of Medical Ethics* (New York: Basic Books, 1981).

7. H. Tristram Engelhardt, Jr. and Michael A. Rie, "Morality for the Medical-Industrial Complex—a Code of Ethics for the Mass Marketing of Health Care," *New England Journal of Medicine* 319, no. 16 (1988): 1086–1089; and Hugo Tristram Engelhardt, *The Foundations of Bioethics* (New York: Oxford University Press, 1986).

8. Donald Seldin, *Beyond Tomorrow* (New York: Rockefeller University Press, 1977).

9. William F. May, *The Physician's Covenant* (Philadelphia: Westminster Press, 1983).

10. Pope John Paul II, *Redemptor Hominis.*

11. D'Arcy, *Humanism and Christianity*, p. 198.

12. Pope John Paul II, "Apostolic Letter: Salvifici Doloris," *Origins* 13, no. 37 (1984): 609.

13. Alasdair MacIntyre, "Moral Philosophy: What Next?" in *Revisions: Changing Perspectives in Moral Philosophy*, ed. Alasdair MacIntyre and Stanley Hauerwas (Notre Dame, Ind.: University of Notre Dame Press, 1983), pp. 1–15.

14. Anthony Ple, *Duty or Pleasure: A New Approach to Christian Ethics* (New York: Paragon House, 1987); Richard B. Brandt, *A Theory of the Good and the Right* (Oxford: Clarendon Press, 1979).

15. Alasdair MacIntyre, *After Virtue*, 2d ed. (Notre Dame, Ind.: University of Notre Dame Press, 1984), Alasdair MacIntyre, *Whose Justice? Which Rationality?* (Notre Dame, Ind.: University of Notre Dame Press, 1988).

16. Hugo Tristram Engelhardt, *Foundations of Bioethics* (New York: Oxford University Press, 1986).

17. Thomas Merton, *No Man Is an Island* (New York: Harcourt, Brace, 1955), p. 153.

18. Hans Jonas, "Commentary: Response to James M. Gustafson," in *Knowing and Valuing: The Search for Common Roots*, ed. Hugo Tristram Engelhardt and Daniel Callahan (Hastings-On-Hudson, N.Y.: Institute of Society, Ethics, and the Life Sciences, 1980), pp. 203–217.

19. Thomas a'Kempis, *The Imitation of Christ* (Milwaukee: Bruce, 1940), p. 3.

8

The Christian Virtues and Autonomy, Beneficence, and Justice

Prima facie principles as conceived by William Ross[1] and adapted by Tom Beauchamp and James Childress have dominated secular bioethics for three decades.[2] Prima facie principles are principles that are intuitively grasped as guides to conduct unless some overriding, more morally compelling reason exists. To be sure, serious doubts are now arising about their sufficiency or universal applicability in medical ethics. But they remain highly influential and, in our opinion, ought to be reckoned with by any alternative theory or ethics. Depending on how we interpret them, prima facie principles can oblige health professionals to laudable standards of moral performance. One may fairly ask, what more would the theological virtues add to this moral life?

In this chapter we will suggest how the dominant prima facie principles relate to, or are shaped by, the Christian virtues. Do they complement, supplement, or replace the prima facie principles? We shall suggest that the theological virtues do not vitiate the prima facie principles but, instead, raise them to the level of grace through the operation of charity, which is the ordering virtue and principle of Christian life. What specifically does this mean for the three principles of autonomy, beneficence, and justice?

Recall that we have already discussed beneficence extensively in our chapters on charity, the ordering principle of the Christian life, and on compassion and caring, putting charity into action. The fourth prima facie principle, nonmaleficence, is subsumed under the principle of beneficence in a model of Christian virtues in medicine.[3] Consequently, we will not discuss beneficence in its own section in this chapter but refer to it as it relates to Christian autonomy and justice.

AUTONOMY AND CHARITY

Autonomy is the most problematic of the prima facie principles because it is individualistic rather than communal in focus. This is especially true in America, where there is so much emphasis on the individual right of freedom from coercion by others. This is an essential moral and legal right, but it can be overemphasized, particularly in libertarian philosophies where it tends toward social fragmentation of an almost Hobbesian kind. Such an excess emphasis on autonomy would be incomparable with autonomy as construed in terms of the theological virtues we have been discussing in this book.

One of the most important ways to respect human beings is to respect their freedom, i.e., their capacity for self-governance. In a word, this respect is respect for their autonomy. This idea was not foreign to classical or medieval ethics, but its locus was in the human will, whereby the moral agent could command action. Yet this freedom was not seen as absolute in the modern sense of self-determination about the good. It was limited because the will could only choose the good, or what appeared to the intellect as a good. The good, however, resided in the natural order of things. It was not a product of either the intellect or the will. St. Thomas and other commentators on Aristotle and Plato emphasized this point, as had Socrates, who had regarded right thinking—choosing the good—as the essence of the moral life.

In these views, one is not free not to choose the good. Hence, if a poor or even evil choice were made, the explanation would be that the intellect did not properly examine the object or that the object was somehow presented to the will as a good. Furthermore, the natural law, which developed into an ethical theory to undergird virtue theory, required human beings to "act in accordance with their nature." In this sense as well, they were not free to abandon the law of their own nature and construct a moral law unto themselves.

Even as late as Hume and the founding fathers of the United States, human beings were regarded as reasonable entities whose happiness lay in conforming their habits of action to their own natures for the good of society itself. Even the rights built into the U.S. Constitution were regarded by Jefferson as the means whereby individuals would do their duty and citizens would act as they ought to act. Rights were not seen as automatic entitlements so much as the social enablement of individual responsibility, a responsibility grounded in human nature.

A rupture occurred in this sunny view of human nature, this "Smile of Reason," as it was called by Sir Kenneth Clark in his televised series *Civilization*. It gave way during and after the Enlightenment to the social disruption of the political and industrial revolutions, on the one hand, and to an increasingly individualistic cast to ethical theory, on the other.

Kant, like the rationalists before him, argued that individuals must conform to a rule of "right reason," a "categorical imperative," in order to act ethically. This reason, however, lay within the individual nature of the person, not in nature itself. Because of Hume's skepticism, the external lawfulness in nature, the Logos of ancient Greek thought, had been subject to doubt. One could not know nature in and of itself. Because of this, all ethical conduct was done out of duty to one's own nature or for duty's sake. Henry Sidgwick summarizes his viewpoint this way: "There can be no separate rational principles for determining the 'material' rightness of conduct, as distinct from its 'formal' rightness; and therefore that all rules of duty, so far as universally binding, must admit of being exhibited as applications of the one general principle that duty ought to be done for duty's sake."[4]

Autonomy meant something different to Kant than it did to his classical and medieval forebears. With Kant the locus of moral interest shifted from free will and the idea of the good, toward which the will intended, to the act of being free itself as the very definition of being human. Kant enjoined individuals to be free in the sense of self-ruling. But this Kantian notion has been eroded in our times by the loss of confidence in the reasonableness of human beings. Certainly the Holocaust and the two major world wars contributed to this postmodern angst. It continues in the ubiquity of violence and social disruptions and in the pursuit of foreign policies such as mutual assured destruction (MAD). These realities make us wonder with Saul Bellow, who exclaims, "To be sane in an age of madness is itself madness."[5]

For Kant, autonomy means more than personal freedom. It means more than conforming one's will to the good. It also means taking responsibility for one's freedom, acting well precisely because one is a human being. It is responsible freedom. This is also Sartre's view, but "responsibleness" is measured not in Kantian terms of duty but in terms of being free itself. Thus, for Sartre there can be a kind of "forced freedom," as distinct from "accepted, responsible freedom." Forced freedom is that which we did not choose but must face. Being born is a good example. We were forced by physiology to leave the womb. To accept freedom is to face and accept the choices we must make and to do so "authentically," i.e., in accord with our own value system. But Sartrian freedom is an isolated, individualistic freedom without external or objective moral standards.

Another stream of transformation in the classical and medieval idea of freedom came in the seventeenth century with the publication of John Locke's *Second Treatise on Government*.[6] Here freedom was construed in negative rather than positive terms as the right not to be encroached upon by others. By entering a social contract with one's fellows, one gives up some of one's personal powers to rules and to rulers. One, in turn, will be protected against the tyranny of those rulers and fellow citizens when they limit freedom unjustly. In Locke's view, society itself is created by a freely contracted agreement among society's members.

Locke's concept of negative rights is carried to its logical extension in the libertarian philosophy of Robert Nozick.[7] Here the shift is to individual development in isolation from others. There is no community obligation to the losers "in the natural lottery," i.e., the poor, the sick, or the handicapped. The individualistic egoism of this view stands out in relief against the older history of natural rights and duties within a community setting. Alexis de Tocqueville astutely diagnosed this notion of freedom and autonomy: "Individualism is a calm and considered feeling which disposes each citizen to isolate himself from the mass of his fellows and withdraw into a circle of family and friends; with this little society formed to his taste, he gladly leaves the greater society to look after itself."[8]

Robert Bellah has noted that human beings in contemporary society now equate community with an enclave of people with whom we either share a common interest or outlook or share a similar income. Gone is the notion of community as those joined "under God" through mutual support and liberty.[9]

In the last twenty-five years autonomy has superseded beneficence as the first principle of medical ethics. This is the most radical reorientation in the long history of the Hippocratic tradition. As a result, the physician-patient relationship has become more honest, open, and respectful of the dignity of patients. Yet new problems have arisen, as autonomy has been absolutized by some and placed in conflict with the goal of beneficence.[10]

This shift in the locus of decision making is a response to the coalescence of sociopolitical, legal, and ethical forces that make it well-nigh irreversible. The central ethical question today is not whether patient autonomy should be preserved but whether it has any moral limits. Does the principle of autonomy as now construed encompass the full meaning of respect for the dignity of persons? May the tendency to absolutize autonomy defeat some of the purposes for which it has been so vigorously propounded? Is there a deeper source for the principle of autonomy that more fully encompasses the special nuances required in authentic respect for persons? Is there a limit on the negative right to be free from coercion?

We take autonomy to be a capacity for self-rule, a quality inherent in rational beings that enables them to make reasoned choices and actions based on a personal assessment of future possibilities evaluated in terms of their own value systems. On this view, autonomy is a capacity that flows from the fact that humans can think and feel and make responsible judgments about what they deem to be good. It is a moral claim on others to act toward us in such a way that capacity for self-governance can function as fully as circumstances permit.

Possession of the virtue of charity produces a profound modification of the idea of autonomy. This modification recognizes autonomy's importance yet sets it within a framework sensitive to obligations to the community and to God. Thus, it returns today's concept of freedom to the older notion of freedom to do the good. But it also goes beyond reason in enhancing the capacity to recognize and to will the good in a much fuller sense, one revealed by the virtue of prudence and sustained by the virtue of love.

For example, charity, unselfish love of God and neighbor, would not perceive active euthanasia or assisted suicide as necessarily "good" deaths. Autonomy illuminated by charity would recognize the complete sovereignty of God. This means that life is a loving gift from God and that humans are stewards of that gift. The intent to accelerate death by directly implementing the means to accomplish it seems to deny that sovereignty and declares humans as masters, not stewards, of life. This reduces the Gospel invitation to the way of the cross to ridicule. Many persons of faith disagree with this assessment of direct killing, and indeed, Christian churches, including our own, have morally permitted killing under specific circumstances, such as in a just war or in capital punishment or self-defense. The moral problematic is intense about all forms of killing, however. The debate continues. What is important to realize is that autonomy itself, from a Christian perspective, is a limited principle, since it is not coherent with the very notion of creation. A creature has obligations to recognize his or her own limits and to honor the Creator's power over life by not usurping it.

Then, too, charity-illuminated autonomy recognizes the individual as part of a community of living beings, or a family of friends to whom we belong. The whole community is diminished by the death of any of its members. Suffering in this community is not a sadomasochistic command of an evil God but the atoning, reconciling identification of human beings with the sufferings of Christ. Death and suffering are not just problems to be solved by our technology but mysteries that teach all of us about our limits and our connectedness with the universe and with one another. How those we love die and how we ourselves eventually accept the suffering of our dying and death reveal even more strongly our common bonds, the importance of making something of our lives, the irreducible vacuity of many human concerns. In short, most often what the dying need is love and humble service on our part.

Charity-illuminated autonomy would also recognize the obligation to preserve health and nurture the gift of life all around us, not to endanger or abuse it. This is true of the environment as well as for personal life. There is, thus, no absolute freedom to reject treatment that is clearly beneficial unless there is some overriding burden, and persons cannot fail to take preventive measures that are under their control. Briefly put, then, there are obligations that follow from being created and redeemed. The fundamental obligation is to exercise intelligent stewardship over the precious gift of life and health. There is, of course, no obligation to submit to or, on the other hand, to demand futile or disproportionately expensive or burdensome treatment.

Without the Christian virtues and carried to extremes, the morally justifiable claim to autonomy could erode the communality of human existence. Autonomy absolutized leads to moral atomism, privatism, and anarchy. Humans are social animals. They cannot be fulfilled except in social relationships, as Aristotle so wisely pointed out.[11] The community within which the patient resides has moral claims as well. This communitarian dimension of biomedical ethics is in danger of compromise if the current drive for autonomy is not modulated and balanced against the moral claims of other persons and the community.

The antagonism some ethicists see between autonomy and beneficence is mitigated by a Christian medical ethic.[12] This is not to justify medical paternalism, which is too often confused with beneficence, but to assert that respect for persons is, in itself, a requirement of beneficence. For the Christian, this beneficence is necessary to the virtue of charity. Humans must be free because each has worth, each is accountable to God, each must be free to follow his or her conscience in moral choices—medical or otherwise.[13]

Viewed from a Christian and Catholic perspective, however, autonomy is not absolute. The Christian is obliged to use his or her God-given freedom wisely and well. Autonomy is a necessary means to doing the right and the good, to fulfilling the stewardship of our own health. This means refraining from self-destruction by suicide, a deleterious lifestyle, or the neglect of needed and appropriate medical care. But if a patient refuses to acknowledge these duties, the physician cannot impose them. Strong paternalism is uncharitable because freedom to choose and shape one's own life is intrinsic to being human. To ignore it is to violate the very humanity of the patient, a humanity given by God.

In the same way, the patient and his or her family have an obligation in charity to respect the autonomy of the health professional or institution. The patient cannot, in the name of the absoluteness of autonomy, demand that the physician become the unquestioning instrument of the patient's will. The conscience of the religious physician or hospital cannot be overridden, even if certain practices such as abortion, sterilization, discontinuance of food and hydration, or euthanasia are legally sanctioned. The Christian, for example, could not accept the absolutization of patient autonomy and self-governance over life so forcefully promulgated by Judge Compton in his concurring opinion in the *Bouvia* case[14] or as argued by Engelhardt in his treatment of the "foundations of bioethics."[15]

The community, too, has a claim to integrity, i.e., to the same kind of wholeness, completeness, and intactness to which the individual lays claim. The fabric of a society can be torn, and the existence of society itself threatened, if individuals retreat into private morality independent of the community. We are in some danger of this when individuals or groups with special interests irresponsibly use resources common to all. Economically, the entrepreneur threatens the integrity of society when he or she despoils the environment. To a certain degree so do physicians, patients, or families who demand and use scarce medical resources when treatment is futile or the benefits disproportionate to the costs.

Patients, therefore, owe a debt to the community for the lifelong benefits they derive from being members of human communities. They should feel some duty to limit their demands for expensive or marginally beneficial treatments and technologies that impose financial burdens on society and their families. Out of a sense of social justice, voluntary limitations should be placed on life-support measures that are futile or that merely prolong the act of dying.

On some of the naturalist views of autonomy, and even beneficence, the physician could be accused of moral abandonment if he or she does not do what the patient thinks is in the patient's own best interests. After all, it is argued, it is the patient who decides what is consistent with his or her own values. Why should the doctor impose on the patient, or frustrate the patient's autonomous decision making? Moreover, is it truly a beneficent act for a physician to refuse a patient's request, especially if the patient is being treated by that physician in a terminal state? Is not the physician bound to assist all patients who suffer to as peaceful a death as possible? Yet ironically, euthanasia as practiced in the Netherlands does not proceed so much from the principle of autonomy as from a balance between the patient's wishes and the physician's own commitment to relieve that patient of suffering. If the physician does not agree with euthanasia in principle, or even if he or she does agree in principle but believes that this particular patient does not qualify, then the physician can deny the request.

Thus, the physician is not bound in the covenant with the patient always to respect that patient's autonomy, although most of the time this is the case. Rather, the physician is bound to respect the personhood of the patient as that personhood develops through its challenges from illness and disease.

The Christian physician's answer to relief of suffering must be a qualified yes. And this is of the utmost importance. The patient's request is not an absolute. Autonomy is only a prima facie principle. It can be overridden by other moral constraints, not the least of which is the physician's own conscience. The request need not be honored, even in painful and dire circumstances, if the patient asks for something that the believing physician considers intrinsically wrong. If this can be so for Dutch physicians who, though convinced of the morality of direct euthanasia, refuse many more patients than they accept, then it surely must be true for a physician who might compassionately suffer along with the patient but draw the line on direct killing as an immoral act under any circumstance. On this Christian view, moved by the Christian virtues of faith, hope, and charity, the patient's life itself is a gift from God over which neither the physician nor the patient can claim dominion or supremacy.

Justice

An essential element of our religious tradition regarding human rights is the understanding that the works of mercy and the works of justice are inseparable. — U.S. Bishops Pastoral Letter on Health and Health Care.[16]

Justice occupies a central place in both principle- and virtue-based theories of ethics. It is one of the cardinal virtues mentioned in Hebrews 8:4, Plato, Aristotle, and the Stoics. Today, it is one of the prima facie principles of medical ethics[17] and central to one of the most influential theories of ethical justification and political liberalism.[18] The relationship of the natural virtue of justice to the theological virtue of charity is especially important for any consideration of the ethics of the Christian health professional or health care institution.

Justice is at the heart of current secular and religious debates about allocation of health care resources. Concerns about justice also include issues such as the mutual obligations of physicians and patients and discrimination in medical-school admission. Both as a principle and as a virtue, justice is a normative concept common to almost every school of ethics, philosophical or theological. For some, it is the pivotal virtue, ordering the other virtues and principles much as charity orders them in Christian ethics.

It is far too ambitious to attempt here even a cursory review of the idea of justice. As a principle or virtue, it has been debated over the centuries.[19] We shall limit our discussion to Plato's and Aristotle's views for the purely philosophical notion and to Thomas Aquinas for the philosophical notion interpreted in the light of Christian revelation. We must also delimit this very large subject to its application in medical ethics.[20]

Plato and Socrates, as Plato depicts him in *The Republic*, review most of the construals of the idea of justice held by their contemporaries.[21] In a series of dialogues—with Polemarchus, Thrasymachus, and Cephalus in book 1 and with Glaucon and Adeimantus in book 2—a wide variety of notions are displayed. Definitions of justice are proposed and critically examined: giving each his due, telling the truth, paying back what is owed, helping friends and harming enemies, an advantage of the strong, and simplicity and goodness of heart. Each definition on closer scrutiny proves to be deficient in one way or another. The quest continues throughout *The Republic* with no unequivocal definition resulting. Nonetheless, justice is identified as a virtue proper to humans, connected with their happiness, and concerning their relationships to each other.

In his characteristically more didactic fashion, Aristotle defines justice as a virtue, an excellence "in relation with his fellow man."[22] Further, he defines the just man as one who, "when making distributions between himself and another, or between two others, will not give himself the larger and his neighbor the smaller share of what is desirable (and vice versa in distributing what is harmful), but . . . will give an equal share as determined by proportion, and he will act the same way in distributing between two others."[23]

As Yves Simon points out, Aristotle was a little obscure in distinguishing the different kinds of justice.[24] Simon's classification of Aristotle's text divides justice into four types: general justice refers to the relation of the members of a community to the whole community; distributive justice, to what the community owes its members according to need and merit; commutative justice, to what members of the community owe each other in their individual relationships; and rectificatory justice, to what the community owes its members when the rules of just exchange between and among members have not been just.

Aquinas' conception of justice as a virtue follows Aristotle in focusing on relationships with others: "It is proper to justice, among other virtues, to direct the human person in those things which pertain to another. For it introduces a certain equality . . . equality is, however, toward another."[25] Aquinas' construal of justice interprets equality in the communal and the individual realms, i.e., the equality of all individuals insofar as they are protected from harm and from coercion that restricts the individual's freedom to pursue natural happiness and fairness in dealing with others.[26] Communal and individual justice are mutually reinforcing and not contradictory. A just society nurtures the fulfillment of the lives of its members, and members of a society become just by fulfilling their obligations to the community. The welfare of the individual is a component of the welfare of the community. Thus, justice is the virtue that disposes humans to respond to the claims of others for equality of treatment—as individuals and as members of a larger whole. As a virtue, it disposes us habitually to respond to needs beyond our own interests and to do so in a fair and equitable way.

The theological virtue of charity also disposes us to respond to needs beyond our own interests. But it does so with a purity of intent and a degree of unselfish love only God's grace can make possible. The Christian thus is inspired to justice, but justice modulated by charity—a charitable justice.

CHARITABLE JUSTICE

Justice, like beneficence, is transformed by the Christian experience of faith in the light of revelation. The pagan notion of justice, like that of the contemporary theories, is ultimately practical and prudential. We owe others their due because we want them to give us our due and because we want to protect ourselves from the unjust claims of others. Justice is a requirement for a peaceable society and the protection of legitimate self-interests. If we practice justice, we thereby can assure happiness for all. Justice, in this view, is a claim we have on the community, compliance with which is an obligation of communal living. In its highest expressions, it might be justified as owed to humans because they are worthy of respect and dignity.

On the Christian view, however, justice has its deepest roots in love; it is an extension of the charity we should show to others. Not to do justice would be to relapse into self-interest, to turn from love of the other to love of self. Love, charity, *caritas, agapē*—each notion testifies that the claims of others upon us are the claims of our brothers and sisters in Christ, loved equally by him and redeemed by him, and thus entitled to be loved.

On the Christian view, therefore, love generates and transmutes justice. As St. Augustine held, justice is the concern and love that Christians must show to others. Charity is for him "the root of all good."[27] It truly is the force moving us to justice. Jesus dedicated his life to justice energized by a love that transcended the legalistic justice of the Pharisees. In the Sermon on the Mount, Jesus calls his disciples to follow him and live not only the letter but the spirit of the Law. His own life is the exemplification of the new justice. St. Paul repeats this exhortation when he calls upon us to put on the "new man."[28]

In his own life, Jesus' concern, his practice of justice transmuted by charity, was for the poor, the sick, the troubled, the oppressed, and the outcast. He practiced justice transmuted by charity in concrete acts of beneficence towards specific persons. He did not argue for charity and justice in conformity with abstract principles. Christian justice does not focus on strict interpretations of what is owed in accordance with some calculus of claims and counterclaims. Instead, it offers the way of love illuminated by an ineffable guide. Christian justice does not obliterate the pagan virtue but modulates and illuminates it by a principle of a very different sort, the principle of charity.[29] It is not knowledge that generates justice, as in Plato or Aristotle, but the loving concern of charity. Jesus on the cross asked the Father to forgive his crucifiers. He did not ask for the retributive justice of the Old Law.

The ways the classical construals of justice in Plato, Aristotle, and the Roman Stoics intersect with the Christian notion are worthy of continuing examination. The same is true of the intersections with contemporary ethics. William Frankena, for example, suggests that the ethics of Christian charity is a theory of its own—"pure agapeism."[30] Justice philosophically derived and justice Christocentrically revealed cannot fully be equated. Their relationships and differences merit closer study in any attempt to answer whether and how Christian notions of love and justice modify the ethics of health care. Just how the natural and supernatural virtues complement, supplement, or transform each other is a subject of its own.[31]

On the Christian view, justice is ultimately grounded in love—a charitable justice rendering to others their due, in which "due" is not only what is legalistically owed but what is called for by love. Charity is the first principle of Christian justice: "There is no limit to love's forbearance, to its trust, its hope, its power to endure."[32] It could be argued similarly on philosophical grounds that justice is ultimately rooted in benevolence and beneficence. In this way, love can be the first principle of naturalistic as well as Christian ethics.

Whether the Christian takes the Augustinian agapeistic, the Thomistic natural-law, or the Christian existentialist perspective, one thing is undeniable—each Christian must respond personally to the life, way, and truth of Jesus Christ. The richness of that truth and its call to perfection are the wellsprings into which Christians must dip for inspiration. This is not to expunge reason but to require that reason confront the unexpungeable reality of Christ's life and teaching. It is in this teaching that we find the ordering force behind Christian justice and love. It is the illuminating power of Christ's healing that becomes the obligation binding Christians to practice a special kind of love and justice.

The awareness of God's call to all to live a life of charity and the conscious answer to this call transform a profession into a vocation. This does not mean that high orders of love and justice are not discernible to non-Christians or that Christians automatically practice these virtues. Indeed, the sad fact is that many do not. Rather, the Christian vocation means fidelity to a notion of justice transmuted by charity. That is a call for every Christian. Health care is one very appropriate response to this call.

Charitable self-effacement is implicit in a Christian vocation to the health ministry. It leads the physician away from a series of activities at the moral margin—things neither illegal nor contravened by professional codes but nonetheless fraught with compromises of Christian conceptions of charity and justice. As we suggested in earlier chapters, we refer here to most of the practices associated with today's commercialism, with competitive and entrepreneurial medicine, e.g., investing in the health care "industry," owning shares in hospitals and nursing homes, patenting medical procedures, and working in for-profit or corporately owned hospitals, clinics, and HMOs. The list of health care investment opportunities open to physicians grows daily. The profit motive sooner or later must conflict with the deference owed the sick person by virtue of the inequality of a relationship in which one of the parties is ill and dependent upon the other. Making a profit from the sickness of others in order to produce a return to investors comes too close to exploitation, even in the best circumstances. This constitutes our objection to Engelhardt and Rie's argument that entrepreneurship is completely ethical.[33]

The Christian is exhorted in the Gospels to "hunger after justice." This means more than fidelity to the natural virtue of justice as taught by Plato, Aristotle, or the Stoics. The Christian is called not only to the natural virtues but also to sanctity, to be perfect "as the Father is perfect," to cooperate with God in God's work. Charitable justice is not content with rights only. It recognizes claims upon us that have no grounding in legal rights but derive from a conception of the human community that enjoins the more fortunate to help the less fortunate whether they "deserve" it or not. There is thus a certain built-in tension between the strictly legal and the Christian senses of justice.

Aquinas examined this tension carefully in his discussion of God's justice and mercy. Replying to the objection that mercy and justice are in contradiction, he said, again, "God's mercy works above his justice, not against it."[34] This is so, Aquinas further says, because God pardons us and a pardon is a "sort of present," something beyond strict justice.

This is a view of justice tempered by mercy, a justice shaped by charity, which looks beyond what is strictly owed arithmetically, economically, or in other human terms. Justice is no longer the pagan goddess, blind, imperturbable, immutable, and absolute in her weighing of the scales. This is the transformation the theological virtue of love works on the natural virtue of justice.

Some of the characteristics of charitable justice become clear when we examine justice in health care delivery. In a strictly legal sense, it is difficult to justify a moral claim by the poor or the sick on the resources of individuals or society. Even more difficult to counter is the argument that the virtuous and the hardworking should sacrifice for the poor, outcasts, sociopaths, alcoholics, or those who abuse their own health.

Yet it is precisely to these groups that Christians, and specifically Catholic Christians, are expected to exercise a "preferential option."[35] The recent pastoral letter of the American bishops and the social encyclicals of the popes since Leo XIII make this clear.[36] When the natural virtue of justice is formed by charity, it goes beyond a strict calculus of duties and claims and is tempered by compassion. Charitable justice gives freely, lovingly, and without respect to strict accounting, which it leaves to God.

One example of how a Catholic Christian perspective might function is in the selection of a principle of distribution when health care resources are scarce, as in the case of kidneys for transplantation, intensive-care beds, or technical procedures of great expense. Distribution theoretically could be on the basis of merit, desert, societal contribution, ability to pay, need, first come first served, lottery, or equity.[37] Of these criteria, merit, desert, societal contribution, and ability to pay are least consistent with the requirements of charitable justice. They suggest measuring a claim to health care in some objective way. On the other hand, equity, need, or perhaps a lottery would be a more suitable response to the vulnerability, plight, and suffering of the sick. Moreover, charitable justice requires that the underlying conditions that lead to rationing choices be eliminated or ameliorated. These conditions cannot be left to the impersonal workings of the marketplace, as so many suggest today. In a Christian community, health care is a communal obligation. To care for the sick is an ordinance of charity, because a caring community is impossible if the suffering of its members is ignored or depreciated.

The ethics of business as it is presently understood cannot therefore be relied upon to guarantee that the extra measure of solicitude that a religious ministry to the sick requires. The Christian physician has a positive responsibility to resist, and even at times to refuse to participate in, actions that endanger patients or treat them discriminatorily out of motives of fiscal necessity. The "economic transfer," for example, of the emergency room patient whose insurance is insufficient to pay for care in a private institution is an example. The ethical dilemmas for conscientious physicians cannot be dissolved by pleading that it is hospital policy or necessary for fiscal survival.

Equally inconsistent with charitable justice is the practice of refusing to see certain patients because of their inadequate insurance. In the same vein, excessive fees, overutilization of diagnostic or therapeutic services, exuberant advertising, maneuvers to dominate the market, and a whole host of morally marginal business practices would be eschewed by physicians who claim Christian authenticity for their ministry to the sick. The physician's "right" to treat whom he pleases would, in a Christian view of medical ethics, be limited by the requirement of justice charitably interpreted.

Another form of behavior antithetical to the Christian notion of love and justice is the refusal to treat certain kinds of patients who represent a threat to the physician. This is true especially of AIDS patients. More and more physicians, nurses, and other health professionals avoid caring for these patients. Some even take the view that AIDS patients are victims of their own self-abuse and not worthy of care. Similar attitudes are evident toward alcoholics, smokers, the very obese, and diabetics who do not follow their dietary regimens.

In short, a Christian vocation of healing imposes a standard of commutative and distributive justice weighed heavily in the direction of benevolence and beneficence even at the expense of inconvenience, cost, and some personal danger to the physician. Simple nonmaleficence does not suffice. Such an interpretation of beneficence is, of course, not closed to the non-Christian. It is often exhibited by those without the Christian imperatives, to the scandal of Christian physicians. But for the Christian, such behavior is a matter of the authenticity of one's faith, of one's response to God's call to healing as a vocation. The Christian physician or health professional cannot live a life of contradiction in which professional and personal morality are divorced. Such a state is inconsistent with even the most rudimentary interpretations of authentic Christian living, to say nothing of a Christian vocation.

In the realms of distributive and social justice a Christocentric ethic would, of necessity, favor some interpretations of justice over others. Thus, Nozick's fundamental principle of protecting the inequalities of the natural lottery would be the antithesis of a Christian perspective. The Christian vocation is oriented quite specifically to a charitable redress of the inequities of the natural lottery. It is, in fact, precisely to the "losers" in the natural lottery—the sick, the poor, the outcast—that Christ addressed his personal ministry, his healing miracles, and his Sermon on the Mount. This is the basis for the preferential option for the poor that inspires the best Christian institutions. These institutions try to practice the good news of the Kingdom of God.

Likewise, distribution of goods and rationing on principles of social worth, merit, productivity, ability to pay, age, or burden on society would be hard to justify. Egalitarian principles of justice, such as Rawls', would have much more claim on the Christian, though not for the reason Rawls adduces—that is to say, not because we ourselves might be the disadvantaged person. Rather, the Christian should show love and justice to all equally, because all are our brothers and sisters under God, not because we might need help ourselves someday. Charitable justice is justice relaxed by mercy, and as such, it reaches out even to those whose own behavior is the cause of their illness or insolvency. The good Samaritan did not inquire into the social history of the traveler he rescued. A Christocentric conception of justice in health care would preclude the physician practicing retributive justice—denying health care because of past abuses of one's health.

Compensatory justice, however, makes amends for injustices in the past. In health care, it would call for extra solicitude for the poor, for minorities, for those who have not had access to health care, and for those badly treated by the natural lottery. It is applicable, too, in admission criteria to medical schools and in such areas as faculty and hospital appointments. On the Christian view, compensatory justice is an obligation implicit in the call to perfection. A preferential option for the poor, the disadvantaged—for all who have been ill-favored by history, environment, heredity, or political or social circumstance—is a necessary extrapolation of justice when it is transformed by Christian charity.

In the realm of social justice, the Christian vocation to health care is a call to the entire community to design and operate institutions and policies that would result in a just and equitable distribution of health care as well as other socially important services. This calls for a united effort on the part of individual health professionals, the health professions as corporate entities, and the entire Christian community. The provision of just and merciful health care to all is thus a shared responsibility in social justice of all Christians. It is not something the laity can delegate to the institutional Church. Collective advocacy for the sick, in all its dimensions, is also a Christian responsibility. The Christian and other religious communities will always be the safety net in a society that tends to accept inequality and two-level medical care as justifiable.

These implications of the charitable concepts of distributive and social justice are not widely acknowledged by Catholics or other Christians. Too many delegate their own responsibility to health professionals, health care institutions, or governmental or voluntary agencies. But all Christians share a mutual responsibility to assure that health care institutions, Catholic-Christian or secular, in fact do act with justice and love. As members of democratic societies, we are expected to use the means available in these societies to shape our institutions. Those who are Christians and bureaucrats have a special vocation to work within their institutional contexts to shape their policies and operations in morally justifiable ways.

Distributive and social justice are most fitting expressions of charitable justice, for Christ provided so many examples of solicitude for the sick that the healing ministry is an essential part of the evangelical ministry of the whole church. Pope John Paul II has recently reaffirmed the importance of that ministry. He reaffirms the good Samaritan parable as a model for Christians, who should be impelled by love and justice to engage in the health care apostolate.[38]

Today, religious hospitals everywhere are tempted by fiscal exigencies to retreat from the care of the poor, to sell out to for-profit corporations, or to compromise with the commercialization and monetarizing practices adopted by their "competitors" and enter into questionable joint ventures and networks. Yet it is precisely the ubiquity and the noncompassionate nature of many of today's accepted practices in hospital finance that generate an ever greater need for continued involvement of the institutional church. Healing always has been essential to the church's evangelical mission. It is also one of the most powerful ways to give public witness to the difference it makes to append the word "Christian" to what we do.

Religious hospitals and health care institutions can compete in today's health care milieu without compromising moral integrity.

They *must* do so to remain faithful to the call we all share to care for the sick.[39] Survival, so much discussed by religious professionals and hospital boards of trustees, cannot include a compromise of justice or a capitulation to practices of dubious ethical nature. This necessitates cooperation in the concrete practice of charity among Catholic and Christian hospitals—a source of economic and moral power still largely neglected. This will call for greater personal and financial support by laypersons and greater volunteer assistance, on a scale not yet practiced. By uniting in the care of the sick, the poor, and the dependent members of a society, Christians demonstrate the indispensability of charitable justice in any human society. This is a message easy to repudiate when preached in the abstract, but difficult to ignore when witnessed in action. It is a message vital to today's world, where every force seems to favor indifference, bureaucratization, commercialization, and depersonalization in caring for the sick. Communities cannot survive without something they love in common, some things that transcend the uninhibited self-interest of the competitive spirit.

All Christians have a vocation—a call from God to follow Christ, "to proclaim the exploits of God who called us out of darkness into this marvelous light."[40] Within this larger call, each person also is called to follow Christ in some specific activity. Whatever that activity may be—exalted or humble—it becomes illuminated by the light of faith and love. "Everyone has his own vocation in which he has been called; let him keep to it."[41]

For the Christian health professional—doctor, nurse, dentist, or other health worker—it is not sufficient to remain faithful to the moral imperatives of a philosophical or naturalistic ethic. A Christian vocation includes the obligations assumed by other professionals, but they must be supplemented by a Christocentric ethic flowing from the Gospel imperatives and other Judeo-Christian revelation, enriched and made congruent with the spirit of a justice transmuted by love. In a vocation, the seminal principles of beneficence and justice central to philosophical ethics are interpreted in the light of the spirit of Sacred Scripture and religious tradition.

CONCLUSION

Pope Paul VI succinctly and eloquently summarized what is essential to a Christian vocation of healing based in love and justice in an allocution he gave to physicians about the profession of medicine:

> Love your profession! It is for you a great school. It sensitizes you to the suffering of your brothers, it helps you to understand and respect them, it purifies the most noble impulses of your heart by the devotion and spirit of self-sacrifice it requires of you. Further, your activity is a great lesson for the whole of society; for it is besides and always the example of generous kindness towards brothers that, more than every word, moves the coldest hearts and offers the life of the community a cause for confidence and moral stability.
>
> How much easier, more beautiful, and more meritorious it is when aid comes to human suffering through the love of Christ, the great mysterious patient who suffers in each of those whom your profession attends with kindness and discernment. (Translation by E. D. Pellegrino)[42]

Paul VI's vision of a Christian profession fuses the idea of profession indissolubly with the idea of vocation. His call is one to which each Christian health professional must respond in the measure of God's grace and as his or her other capabilities allow. It is a vision that the committed Christian will grasp.

In Christian life, the virtues shape the individual and the community toward an ideal of perfection.[43] In a secular ethics model, there is less of a sense of development toward a goal, since one starts with the ideal already—respect for the autonomy of each person in the dialogue.[44] Inevitably, then, there is a conflict for the Christian physician in the method of analysis of moral issues that underlies the adoption of a secular bioethics. For the most part, we are able to reach accommodation with the well-rehearsed principles of modern bioethics, since they make sense in a secular, pluralistic environment. Moreover, many Christian physicians will disagree about the exact place to draw the line on certain actions. This is a function of the uniqueness of our upbringing and experiences in life. This is only natural. The challenge is to be persuasive to a larger society about the commitments and obligations this loving ethic requires. We attempt that next in our last chapter.

NOTES

1. William David Ross, *The Right and the Good* (Indianapolis/Cambridge: Hackett, 1988).

2. Tom L. Beauchamp and James F. Childress, *Principles of Biomedical Ethics*, 4th ed. (New York: Oxford University Press, 1994).

3. We leave aside the fourth, nonmaleficence. We agree with Beauchamp and Childress that nonmaleficence is also a prima facie principle, but for us it is a minimalist principle that, for our present purposes, can be regarded as the negative formulation of the principle of beneficence.

4. Henry Sidgwick, *Outlines of the History of Ethics* (Indianapolis: Hackett, 1988), pp. 272–273.

5. Saul Bellow, *Henderson, the Rain King* (New York: Viking Press, 1959).

6. John Locke, *Second Treatise on Government*, 3d ed. (Oxford: Basil Blackwell, 1966).

7. Robert Nozick, *Anarchy, State, and Utopia* (New York: Basic Books, 1974).

8. Alexis de Tocqueville, *Democracy in America* [Vol. 2], trans. George Lawrence, ed. J. P. Mayer (New York: Doubleday, Anchor Books, 1969), p. 506.

9. Robert N. Bellah et al., *Habits of the Heart: Individualism and Commitment in American Life* (New York: Harper and Row, 1986).

10. Edmund D. Pellegrino and David C. Thomasma, *For the Patient's Good: The Restoration of Beneficence in Health Care* (New York: Oxford University Press, 1988).

11. Aristotle, *Politics*, trans. Benjamin Jowett (New York: Modern Library, 1943), 1253a (25–30), p. 55.

12. For a secular view of the clash, see Tom L. Beauchamp and Lawrence McCullough, *Medical Ethics: The Moral Responsibilities of Physicians* (Englewood Cliffs, N.J.: Prentice-Hall, 1984).

13. Walter M. Abbott, ed., *The Documents of Vatican II* (London: Geoffrey Chapman, 1962).

14. *Bouvia v. Superior Court of the State of California for the County of Los Angeles* (Glenchur), 179 Cal. App. 3d 1127, 225 Cal. Rep. 297 (Ct. App. 1986); Review denied (Cal. June 5, 1986).

15. H. Tristram Engelhardt, Jr., *The Foundations of Bioethics* (New York: Oxford University Press, 1986).

16. U.S. Bishops Council, "Pastoral Letter: On Health and Health Care," *Origins* 11, no. 25 (1981): 396–402.

17. Beauchamp and Childress, *Principles of Biomedical Ethics*.

18. John Rawls, *A Theory of Justice* (Cambridge: Harvard University Press, 1971); and *Political Liberalism* (New York: Columbia University Press, 1993).

19. See the discussion and bibliography in *The Great Ideas: A Symposium of Great Books of the Western World*, ed. Mortimer Adler and William Gorman (Chicago: Encyclopedia Britannica, 1952), pp. 850–879.

20. See also our discussion of the natural virtue of justice in Edmund D. Pellegrino and David C. Thomasma, *The Virtues in Medical Practice* (New York: Oxford University Press, 1993), chapter 8, pp. 92–108.

21. Plato, *The Republic of Plato*, trans. Allan Bloom (New York: Basic Books, 1968).

22. Aristotle, *Nicomachean Ethics*, trans. Martin Ostwald (Indianapolis: Bobbs-Merrill/Liberal Arts Press, 1962), 1129b: 26, 26, p. 99.

23. Aristotle, *Nicomachean Ethics*, 1134a: 2-6, p. 128.

24. Yves R. Simon, *The Definition of Moral Virtue* (New York: Fordham University Press, 1986), pp. 99–100.

25. St. Thomas Aquinas, *Summa Theologiae* [Vol. 37], trans. Thomas Gilby (New York: Blackfriars, 1975), II-II, q. 57, a. 1, pp. 2–7; and *Summa Theologiae* [Vol. 23], trans. William D. Hughes (New York: Blackfriars, 1969), I-II, q. 60, a. 2, pp. 100–103.

26. Jean Porter, *The Recovery of Virtue: The Relevance of Aquinas for Christian Ethics* (Louisville: Westminster/John Knox Press, 1990), p. 136.

27. St. Augustine, Sermon 72.4, in *Fathers of the Church,* as cited by William J. Walsh and John P. Langan, "Patristic Social Consciousness—The Church and the Poor," in *The Faith That Does Justice*, ed. John C. Haughey (New York: Paulist Press, 1977), p. 118.

28. Romans, chap. 6, in *The New American Bible* (New York: Catholic Book Publishing, 1970), pp. 185–186.

29. The question about the continuity or discontinuity of the supernatural and the natural virtues is still an intriguing one. Robert Sokolowski has examined this relationship in a brilliant monograph, illuminating both kinds of virtue: *The God of Faith and Reason* (Notre Dame: University of Notre Dame Press, 1982).

30. William Frankena, *Ethics*, 2d ed. (Englewood Cliffs, N.J.: Prentice-Hall, 1973).

31. Sokolowski, *God of Faith and Reason*.

32. 1 Corinthians 13:1–8, in *The New American Bible*, pp. 206–207.

33. H. Tristram Engelhardt, Jr. and Michael A. Rie, "Morality for the Medical-Industrial Complex—A Code of Ethics for the Mass Marketing of Health Care," *New England Journal of Medicine* 319, no. 16 (1988): 1086–1089.

34. St. Thomas Aquinas, *Summa Theologiae* [Vol. 5], trans. and ed. Thomas Gilbey (New York: Blackfriars, 1973), I, q. 21, a. 3, pp. 78–81.

35. Charles E. Curran and Richard A. McCormick, eds., *Readings in Moral Theology No. 2: The Distinctiveness of Christian Ethics* (New York: Paulist Press, 1980); and *Readings in Moral Theology No. 5: Official Catholic Social Teaching* (New York: Paulist Press, 1986).

36. U.S. Catholic Conference, *Catholic Social Teaching and the U.S. Economy: Health and Health Care: A Pastoral Letter of the American Catholic Bishops* (Washington: U.S. Catholic Conference, 1981).

37. W. Norman Pittenger, *Catholic Faith in a Process Perspective* (Maryknoll, NY: Orbis, 1981).

38. Pope John Paul II, *Apostolic Letter: Salvifici Doloris* (Washington: U.S. Catholic Conference, 1984).

39. Edmund D. Pellegrino, "Catholic Hospitals: Survival without Moral Compromise," *Health Progress* 66, no. 4 (1985): 42–49.

40. 1 Peter 2:9, in *The New American Bible*, p. 281. See "Vocation," in *A Catholic Dictionary*, ed. D. Attwater, 2d ed. (New York: Macmillan, 1949), p. 520.

41. 1 Corinthians 7:20, in *The New American Bible*, p. 201.

42. Paul VI, "Allocution a des medecins," in *Documents pontificaux de Paul VI* (St. Maurice, Switzerland: Editions Saint-Augustin, 1970), p. 701:

> Aimez votre profession! Elle est pour vous une grande école. Elle vous sensibilise a la souffrance de vos freres, elle vous aide à les comprendre et à les respecter, elle purifie les plus nobles élans de votre coeur par le devouement et l'esprit de sacrifice qu'elle exige de vous. Votre activite est encore une grande lecon pour la societe tout entiere: car c'est encore et toujours l'example de la bonte genereuse envers ses freres qui mieux que toute parole, entraine les ames, emeut les coeurs les plus froids, et offre à la vie de la communaute un motif de confiance et de stabilite morale. Combien elle est plus facile, plus belle, plus meritoire lorsqu'elle vient en aide a la souffrance humaine par amour du Christ, le grand Patient mysterieux, qui souffre en chacun de ceux sur lesquels se penche avec bonte et discernement votre profession.

43. Roberto Cessario, *The Moral Virtue and Theological Ethics* (Notre Dame: University of Notre Dame Press, 1991).

44. H. Tristram Engelhardt, Jr., *Bioethics and Secular Humanism* (Philadelphia: Trinity Press International, 1991).

9

The Christian Personalist Physician

What I feel like telling you today is that the world needs real dialogue, that falsehood is just as much the opposite of dialogue as is silence, and that the only possible dialogue is the kind between people who remain what they are and speak their minds. This is tantamount to saying that the world of today needs Christians who remain Christians.[1]

—Albert Camus, "The Unbeliever and Christians"

Up to this point our book has attempted to define the Christian virtues of faith, hope, and charity and to show how they modify the practice of medicine and the healing professions and the ethical principles of beneficence, autonomy, and justice. But principles and virtues, whether theological or philosophical, do not exist as concepts alone. If they are to be existentially as well as essentially linked, they must be synthesized in human persons. This is why we commented so frequently that the standards of virtue ethics are not just an ideal existing in some world of perfection. *Aretē*, perfection, is refracted through in the role models of individual humans living in community with each other.

The ethics of virtue—that is, the formation of the good person in a good society—dominated moral philosophy through most of its history. It still commands pride of place in religious ethics. But as MacIntyre has so cogently demonstrated, virtue ethics has come gradually to be superseded by a more rationalist form of ethics. Virtue ethics depends on a consensus about the characteristics of human nature, its ends and purposes. This consensus eroded during and after the eighteenth-century Enlightenment.[2] Instead of concentrating on the good person, on what we should be, ethics came to focus increasingly on the act performed instead.

THE CHRISTIAN PERSON: EMBODIMENT OF VIRTUES AND PRINCIPLES

Persons acting in the here and now are the embodiment of both virtues and principles. They struggle with their choices in concrete circumstances. They take specific actions that have consequences, not only for their lives but also for the lives of many others. These actions are initiated by specific intentions. The moral psychology of Christian ethics can only be expressed in the actuality of the Christian person.

The idea of personhood is not to be found in any explicit way in the Greek philosophers. Personhood is essentially a Christian idea, born in an effort to understand the complexities of redemption by the person of Jesus Christ and his relationship with the Trinity. From its origins in the early church, the concept of person underwent intense development through the Middle Ages, then received further enrichment in our times by insights drawn from contemporary existential and phenomenological philosophies. Let us look at this development briefly.

In Greek philosophy, the concept of person can only be drawn inferentially. For example, at one point in *The Symposium*, Plato refers to that which remains constant in us throughout all the somatic and psychic changes humans experience.[3] This substratum could be interpreted as the person that perdures throughout an individual's life changes. It would be consistent also with Aristotle's teaching about the indivisible unity of body and soul as well as potentiality, actuality, and change. In any case, the idea of person can only be imputed to the philosophies of Aristotle, Plato, and the Stoics. It is not defined precisely in their writings and certainly not in the sense the concept assumed in Christian and medieval philosophy and theology.

For the Romans, persons were juridical entities, those entitled by law to the privilege of citizenship. This entitlement separated Roman citizens from slaves and foreigners. This Roman concept emphasized the person as the bearer of legal rights in much the same way that modern secular notions of personhood often do. This is an impoverished yet partially true notion of person.

Similarly, in Hebrew Scriptures, the idea of person was implicit. Although it is not formally developed, the biblical idea comprised the elements of what in later Christianity would be more explicitly defined as personhood: "You knew me through and through from having watched my bones take shape when I was being formed in secret, knitted together in the limbo of the womb" (Psalm 139). "Your hands molded and made me" (Job 10:8-12). "From my mother's womb you have been my God" (Psalm 22). "Before you were born I set you apart" (Jeremiah 1:4-10).

These scriptural texts speak to a relationship of persons. A personal God addresses, and is addressed by, persons he has created. These are persons God has made, whom He knows, calls, and shapes and from whom he expects responses. God also holds these persons accountable for the ways in which they respond to his call. They are not just individual instantiations of a species but persons who can know, respond, and interact as persons with God and are accountable to him.

From the beginning, the Christian Gospels called individual persons to salvation and made individuals accountable and responsible for accepting or rejecting that call. The Jesus of the Gospels appeals as a person to other persons who are free to follow or reject him as a person. Jesus refers to God as the Father, his Father and ours. The parables tell of the good and the bad, the right and the wrong done by persons free to choose, free to act. The choice and the act are expressions of the person, who is shaped by his or her choice and action.

A more formal theological and philosophical conception of personhood emerged in the fifth and sixth centuries A.D in response to the vigorous debates and the heresies surrounding the question of the personhood of Christ. Most notably, in 451 the Council of Chalcedon rejected the Monophysite heresy[4] by asserting Christ to be one person in two natures. In the milieu of these debates, Boethius (475-524), often called the last of the Roman philosophers and the first of the Scholastics, defined the person as "an individual substance of a rational nature."[5]

In this definition, Boethius recognized, as had Aristotle, the essential unity of body and soul in human beings. Man was an individual thing by virtue of that part of him which was derived from matter. He was a person by virtue of that part of him which derived from spirit. If we deprive humans of their personhood, we reduce them to individual matter, to mere single instances of a species, set apart by the uniqueness of their accidental characteristics but lacking the rational nature on which their personhood depends. Yet persons are not disembodied spirits but spirits in substantial union with bodies.

Boethius' definition was the dominant conception of person for a very long time. Despite the intervening centuries, as a philosophical definition, it has not been improved upon. It captures the essential ontological nature of personhood, although its content has been more fully fleshed out in recent Christian theology, as we shall see shortly. Boethius' definition was the major influence on Christian medieval philosophers, such as Aquinas and Bonaventure, who applied it to the personhood of God.[6] They fused the earlier theological and philosophical construals of personhood. This was consistent with the whole enterprise of Christian medieval philosophy, which was to bring Greek philosophy and Christian revelation into accord with each other.

Since the Middle Ages, the Boethian definition of person has been subjected to different interpretations by successive schools of philosophy. Descartes, Hume, and contemporary phenomenologists and existentialists such as Heidegger, Sartre, Levinas, Buber, and Scheler, to name just a few, have modified and, at times, enriched the Boethian concept.[7] It is impossible to detail these transformations here. But one contemporary construal of personhood is most pertinent to the central theme of this book, and that is the concept of person set forth in the writings of His Holiness John Paul II.

In previous extended work and more recently in his book *Crossing the Threshold of Hope*, the Holy Father outlines a powerful philosophy of Christian personalism.[8] His "personalist principle" is his attempt to "translate the commandment of love into the language of philosophical ethics."[9] In this effort, the Holy Father enriches the rational component of Boethius' metaphysical definition with insights drawn from contemporary phenomenology.[10] The result is a view of humans as acting persons free to transcend nature and to fulfill themselves by giving of themselves in love.

Indeed, the Holy Father says that the "full truth about man" is that he "affirms himself most completely by giving of himself."[11] This is the way persons affirm themselves as persons and fulfill the commandment of love at the same time.[12] This is the central truth of the Christian ethic, expressed in our relation to family, community, and vocation. In these relationships, we are called to use our freedom to give ourselves to others. Not to give oneself to others is to end up giving ourselves only to ourselves and to become selfish. For the selfish person, the good is that which gives him or her pleasure. This desire for total independence in the moral life creates the "inner division of man."[13] Such independence is not true freedom since freedom cannot exist apart from truth.[14]

John Paul II's concept of the person clearly is more than the individual atomism of John Locke's contract theory. Nor can it ever be simply the genetically or environmentally determined "individual" of sociobiology or the politically determined individual of liberal democracy. Although it may draw upon them for certain insights, the concept of person cannot be reduced to anthropology, psychology, or phenomenology. The Christian view of personhood goes beyond the Kantian imperative not to use others merely as means. Rather, the person is to be affirmed as a person, possessing dignity simply because he or she is a person. Man is a personal being, created and loved by a personal God and destined to be united face-to-face with the Creator.

This Christian conception of personhood has clear implications for the nature of the physician's vocation and for the way one pursues that vocation. Let us turn next to these two aspects of the person's acting as physician in relation to patients and in relation to ethical choices.

CHRISTIAN PERSONALISM AND THE CHRISTIAN PHYSICIAN

In these days of high technology, it is ever more difficult to remember that medicine is essentially a relationship of persons. Yet this is what makes it a moral enterprise. This is why medical ethics is unavoidably grounded in some concept of personhood. Ultimately, both the ethics of the patient-physician relationship and the making of ethical decisions depend on our conception of the human person. Despite this, most of bioethics today avoids or trivializes the question of personhood.

But personhood is a question that cannot be avoided. Implicit in every theory and decision of medical ethics is some notion of what it is to be human, of the purposes, ends, and goods of human existence. In secular bioethics, there is an implicit, yet dominant, concept of personhood. As we saw in the previous chapter, personhood is defined in terms of freedom, liberty, self-expression, and self-generated or socially constructed norms of good and evil. The question of ultimate ends or purposes to human life is, at best, laid aside as irrelevant or regarded as a morally neutral item of individual preferences. The possibility of an objective moral order or a source of morality outside humans, individually or collectively, is not part of the discourse. It is relegated to the dustbin of medieval metaphysical eccentricities, too naive for serious consideration in the post modern, post-Christian world.

Christian anthropology stands in opposition to this dominant view. Christian anthropology, as exemplified in the Christian personalism of Pope John Paul II, shapes medical ethics in specific ways.[15] We will look at two ways: (1) professional ethics, which pertains to the obligations of the Christian physician as a physician, and (2) problem-oriented ethics, which pertains to certain specific ethical dilemmas involving human life.

1) Professional Issues

The Christian physician as a human person has the same vocation as all Christian persons: to fulfill oneself in giving oneself to others—to family, friends, neighbors, strangers. In addition, as a physician, the Christian person is called to a special way of love, of giving oneself in one's daily works of healing, helping, curing, and caring. Physicians and patients are persons interacting in a specific existential situation in which one is vulnerable and suffering and seeks healing from another who offers to help and heal. By its nature, the healing relationship is unequal. The patient's personhood is exposed to, and by, the physician—bodily, spiritually, and emotionally. The patient's need for affirmation as a person in the face of this exposure is intense and a source of moral obligation for the physician.

Of course, this is true of the relationship between patients and non-Christian physicians as well. What is different for the Christian physician is that healing is more than an occupation or a career. Healing is a vocation, a call from a personal God to a specific way of giving of oneself to other persons, a specific way of loving, of fulfilling oneself as a person and working toward one's own salvation. This is very different from a career that is an end in itself, in which medicine is cultivated for personal ends and purposes. Every true profession entails some degree of suppression of self-interest.[16] But a vocation is a call by God to transmute a profession into the domain of grace and charity.

What does this mean in everyday practice? It means taking as obligations what others would regard as supererogatory or even heroic. It means a preferential option for care of the poor, the sick, and the rejected. It calls the physician to recognize the dignity of the person in the drug addict, the sociopath, the alcoholic, and the criminal, as well as in the respected members of the community. The hard message of unselfish sacrifice, like the message of the Gospel story of the good Samaritan, becomes the physician's model of healing. The Christian physician, for example, cannot protest that treating AIDS was "not in his contract" when he entered medical school.

For Christians, medicine cannot become a commercial enterprise; the physician, an entrepreneur; or the hospital, a profit-making venture. We cannot ask whether the noncompliant or the self-abusing patient "deserves" medical care. Our model is Christ in the first chapter of Mark, healing all who came to him at the end of the day, never asking the supplicants who or what they were. Christian physicians must be advocates for the sick whenever the interests of the sick person are subverted for economic or political exigency. If managed care calls us to be indifferent to the needs of patients or makes us instruments of economics or profit, we must resist. If managed competition turns us into fund holders, case managers, and clinical economists, we must refuse. Sick persons are not consumers of our product or clients; they are *patients*—persons suffering, bearing an illness, in need of relief that we are called to provide as best we can.

Fidelity to a Christian personalist anthropology transforms the principles that currently dominate secular medical ethics. It shapes them by the ordering principle of charity. Beneficence becomes more than avoiding harm or preventing evil. It comes to mean doing good for others and for patients even when it means the sacrifice of some degree of legitimate self-interest. As Luke 6:36 says, "We must be compassionate as our Father is compassionate." We must feel the personal predicament of illness as it confronts this particular person in all his or her individuality and personhood. Beneficence becomes charitable beneficence, effacement of self-interest for the good of the patient.

For those who fear that suppression of self-interest is unrealistic and ignores legitimate self-interest, we need to remember Aquinas' interpretation of the commandment of love. That command was not to love others as much as we love ourselves, but in the same way as we love ourselves—i.e., by loving others for God's sake, for their intrinsic value, and by meeting their legitimate, not their illegitimate, desires. Effacement of self-interest within these limits is essential to a Christian vocation to medicine[17]

Autonomy becomes more than the Lockean negative right to noninterference. It becomes respect for the inherent dignity of each person as a person, that which is "most perfect in nature" as St.

Thomas put it. In secular use, autonomy has come to mean the right not only to govern one's own life but to determine what is the right life, not what I *ought* to do, but what *I* determine ought to be done. Autonomy must be restored to its original meaning of having to take responsibility for one's choice, rather than making one's choice the standard of right and wrong. We respect autonomy because it is the freedom to do the good and to give oneself, not the freedom to determine what is right or wrong.

Justice, too, is transformed from a strict, rendering of what is merited or owed, to charitable justice. This is justice tempered by mercy. Charitable justice may require giving more than is owed. It measures what is owed in different terms—in terms of love, compassion, and mercy. Charitable justice is not the blind justice of popular iconography. It is justice without the blindfolds, sensitive to those nuances of each person's unique predicament of illness. Charitable justice measures what each person needs by adding that aliquot of mercy which balances the scales in a way demanded by the commandment of love.

When the Christian concept of person underlies the physician-patient relationship, that relationship becomes a relationship of love, not in a sentimental or physical sense but in the sense of giving oneself and one's knowledge for the benefit of others, as Christ would have done. Even practices not positively unethical then become unacceptable—unrelenting pursuit of legitimate fees, impatience, insensitivity, unavailability, inaccessibility, or rudeness, even to difficult patients. In a Christian ethics of vocation to medicine, charity is, of necessity, the ordering and the distinguishing ethical principle and virtue.

The Christian idea of person thus imposes extraordinary responsibility on physicians and institutions that profess to be Christian. Much of what is required is alien to the bureaucratized, industrialized, and depersonalized labyrinth health care has become. The marketplace, the bottom line, and the corporation know nothing of the commandment of love, which John Paul II puts at the center of his personalist ethics. It is the specific vocation of all Christian physicians and institutions to restore this truth about the person to the center of health care today.

If Christian personalism shapes the ethics of the physician-patient relationship in ways antithetical to contemporary trends, so too does it shape the moral choices physicians and society must make in the use of contemporary biotechnology.

2) Personalism and Dilemma Ethics: Human-Life Issues as Examples

In addition to shaping the physician-patient relationship, a Christian anthropology shapes the way clinical decisions are made and clinical dilemmas resolved. This is especially so in the key human-life issues—e.g., abortion, embryo and fetal-tissue research, treatment of the mentally incompetent, withholding and withdrawing life support, and euthanasia. Indeed, the truth about the human person is the only safeguard against a technological imperative that knows no bounds as long as the utility to be gained and the costs to be saved are the ordering principles. A secular bioethics is impotent to prevent the harm to the most vulnerable members of our species inherent, for example, in the misuse of modern reproductive technology or in embryo research or the involuntary or nonvoluntary euthanasia of the handicapped or intellectually retarded.

Abortion is considered an abomination because it destroys a creature created and "molded" in the womb (Psalm 139) by a personal God to be loved by God. This created being is worthy of respect because it is a person on the way to full actualization. Abortion deprives that person of its destiny to be loved and to love. No arbitrary biological marker or time interval can change the fact that the fertilized egg is an individual substance belonging to a species of beings with a rational nature created by a personal God.

This is also the case with embryo and pre-embryo research. The NIH Advisory Panel on Human Embryo Research notwithstanding, embryos must not be created for the purposes of research and then discarded.[18] Nor can a blastomere be used to diagnose genetic defects and be destroyed if they are present. Nor can fetal tissues taken from electively aborted fetuses be used for experimentation or transplantation.[19] A Christian personalist anthropology places clear ethical limits on the use of technology, no matter how useful, important, or profitable it may be.

It is impossible here to provide a critique of the many recommendation of the NIH Advisory Panel on Human Embryo Research. But even a cursory review of the list reveals a total indifference to anything approaching the Catholic Christian concept of personhood. This applies to all three of the panel's categories—"acceptable," "unacceptable," and "research that warrants further review."[20] Given the utilitarian reasoning of the panel members, it is doubtful whether any manipulations of embryos will remain unacceptable for long. As long as the benefits of the research are the deciding factor, the embryo is at risk from almost every kind of manipulation. We must hope that believers and nonbelievers alike will refuse to permit any form of research with human embryos that is not intended for the direct benefit of the particular embryo that is the subject of the research.

The same ethical constraints must be placed on the manifold possibilities of the Human Genome Project.[21] Gene manipulation for therapeutic purposes that benefit the person who is subject to research would be licit. Manipulations aimed at enhancement of certain characteristics such as height, intelligence, or memory are morally bankrupt. Manipulations to remake the human race in accord with some utopian, biologically conceived image of the ideal human person would be totally reprehensible and an affront to God's continuing creative presence in the world.

Increasingly distorted notions of the human person are used to justify proposals that, even a short time ago, would have been thought abominable. For example, one ethicist has suggested that persons in a permanent vegetative state should be used for experimental purposes rather than animals of other species because these "animals" lead less full lives than healthy animals.[22] Others suggest that the retarded and the brain-damaged are mere biological remnants, too costly to sustain in life because they are nonpersons.[23] Active euthanasia and assisted suicide also arise from a contortion of the notion of autonomy such that the person becomes not the creature but the creator of his own life. The State of Oregon has given legal sanction to assisted suicide by permitting physicians to write, and pharmacists to fill, prescriptions for lethal doses of medication.[24]

These challenging trends arise from the failure of secular ethics to confront the question of personhood and its implications, but even more strongly from a grossly disordered notion of personhood as identified only with self-awareness, consciousness, or the ability to establish meaningful social relationships or lead a "quality life" as measured by some standard of idyllic bliss free of all suffering. On the secular view, we lose our dignity if we are sick, in pain, suffering, disfigured, or unable to handle our secretions and excretions without assistance. Often enough, objections to these views are simply framed as counterassertions, without sufficient thought about the nature of personhood and the obligations that necessarily flow from the freedom, moral choices, and consequent power we enjoy over the range of all living organisms.

None of the secular views of persons and suffering can be countered without a true notion of what it is to be a human person, wherein the source of dignity resides. That notion can never be true unless it calls upon the grounding of personhood in God's love for us and his gift of freedom which permits us to give of ourselves to fulfill ourselves. This is the only way pain, suffering, and death can acquire meaning. It is the only genuine source of human dignity, which cannot be lost.

Catholic and Christian physicians today have a mission of the utmost importance to the whole of society. They must, of course, be competent, caring, and compassionate physicians. But they must also know the true ends and purposes of human life, know the truth about the human person for whom they care, and that truth must inform their practice—as physicians—and how they approach health care and the manipulation of human life.

Torn loose from its moorings in Christian anthropology, ethics can eradicate our very existence as human persons. In times past, only despots perpetrated such tragedies. Today, with the erosion and deconstruction of the idea of person, we seem on the verge of legitimating depersonalization, not as an act of despotism but by the sanction of a secularist conception of what it is to be a human person. In this Catholic physicians are under special obligation: first, to give collective and personal witness to the difference it makes to adhere to the truth about the human person; then, to reach out to, and gain the support of, physicians of other faiths to resist the corrosion of the notion of the person that pervades secular bioethics; and, finally, to inform public opinion lest all of humanity be diminished in the name of a false humanism that denies its own roots in the true conception of what it is to be a human person.

OBLIGATIONS TO RESPECT PERSONS IN THE DOCTOR-PATIENT RELATIONSHIP

Our age is strangely paradoxical in its approach to human life. On the one hand, we see an enormous solicitude for individual lives in peril from natural disasters—including the lives of trapped whales. On the other ours is the bloodiest era in human history, encompassing atomic wars, internecine struggles in many countries, violations of human rights by governments, and the unprecedented killing of millions through elective abortion.

On balance, the value of human life has depreciated in our age. Literature, music, and art attest to the tenuous state of our individual lives. Mere survival for many citizens is a major achievement when human life can be neatly obliterated by an interuterine injection of saline, a bullet from a Saturday night special, a drunken driver, a dose of crack, or even the slower dissolution of lung tissue by polluted air or hidden radon gas in our homes.

Against this negative scenario, medicine, by virtue of its central healing intent, must assert respect for human life and human persons. Apart from religious organizations, medicine remains one of the few truly effective forces on the international scene fostering the dignity and value of individual human beings. But in today's antilife environment, the healing enterprise of medicine is in serious jeopardy because of attacks from many directions.[25]

Few would countenance the more direct and brutish assaults on the healing functions of medicine, such as the use of physicians to declare political dissidents insane or to monitor their torture. The more subtle erosions are perhaps the more dangerous—the encouragement of medical entrepreneurship, the legitimation of the profit motive and the rule of the marketplace in health care, the transformation of medicine into applied biology, or the designation of the physician as society's gatekeeper—ordained to protect its resources rather than advocate the needs of the patient. To transform the physician's role into that of bureaucrat, proletarian, businessman, or social engineer is to subvert the ends of medicine, which should center on the well-being of the sick person. Without this center the other roles become odious. Any conflict between the interests of the person the physician attends and other interests must be guarded against assiduously.

Because of these corrosive forces and the subtle as well as the overt temptations to betray the central commitment of medicine to patients, it is essential to reflect on the concept of respect for persons, the general principle from which respect for the personhood of the sick human being derives. It is clear that

1. respect for persons is central both to medicine and to religion;
2. the ethical norms that should guide the conduct of health professionals derive from respect for persons;
3. religious affirmation strengthens these norms in a way that goes beyond what medicine philosophically considered can

deduce and beyond a concept of autonomy alone governing medical-ethical transactions.

What other obligations does a religious point of view bring to caring for the individual patient in the health care setting?

1) Respect for Religious Beliefs

Whatever one's personal beliefs or nonbeliefs, it is an obligation rooted in the principle of respect for persons to know the religious values of the patient. This is obviously the case when the caregiver is making decisions for the patient's benefit. Respecting these values is part of setting up the goals of medical care. They are part of establishing the good of the patient. One must not scoff at or denigrate these beliefs.

If they share these beliefs, the physician can then help the patient to draw upon the spiritual resources available within him or herself, the community of believers, and the faith in order to make authentic decisions.

If they do not share beliefs, the physician must still take these beliefs into account in constructing a value-based therapeutic plan.[26] If a physician finds the beliefs of a patient offensive then he or she must withdraw respectfully from the care of that patient and find a replacement. In this regard, a secular humanist physician has no more right to impose his or her utilitarianism or libertarianism on the patient than does a religious zealot. Respect for persons means just that. It means that a physician would help the patient get spiritual aid if requested or if the physician senses the patient's need for it.

2) The Healing Relationship

In the changed sociopolitical, economic, and scientific climate within which medicine is practiced today, there are conflicting conceptions of the healing relationship. Some of the formulations of this relationship would be more congenial to a Christian perspective than others. Thus, it would not require a high degree of Christian discernment to see that a biological model of the physician-patient or healing relationship would be insufficient, if not antithetic, to a Christian interpretation of healing or helping. The same could be said of the relationship viewed as a legal contract, as a commodity exchange, or as strong paternalisim. Other models—covenant, friendship, or fidelity to promise—would be more congruent.[27]

All the models cited have some verisimilitude. Without denying this fact, it is the model perceived as primary that is of utmost importance, that takes precedence over the others. Thus, strong paternalism would rarely, if ever, be countenanced while weak paternalism could be.[28] A strictly libertarian relationship would not be consistent, since it would forbid intervention in suicide or euthanasia, for example. With these exceptions, respect for the autonomy of the competent patient as a human person would not only be consistent but required. So, too, would respect for the respective agency of patient and physician, with neither imposing on the other except where grave harm was in prospect. There would also be a strong imperative that both physician and the patient have mutual respect for personal moral accountability. Neither could ask the other to act contrary to conscience.

Likewise, a strictly contractual model of the healing relationship is insufficient from a Christian perspective. The contractual model requires only a minimalistic ethic obligating the patient and the physician to fulfill the terms of an agreement and nothing more. This model calls for the minimal amount of beneficence. Rather, it is contrived to reduce dependence upon either the physician's benevolence or fidelity to promises. It is precisely those features of the relationship that a contract cannot cover—the uncertainties inherent in the clinical situation, and reliance on the fidelity and good will of the physician and patient—that charity most clearly regulates.

The most distinctive characteristic of a healing relationship motivated by the Christian perspective is the higher degree of self-effacement it requires as a matter of course. Even on strictly philosophical grounds, the vulnerability of the sick person imposes a special responsibility not to take advantage of the patient. In a more positive sense, physicians commit themselves to some degree of suppression of their own self-interests, comfort, and preferences in order to serve the patient. This "higher degree of self-effacement" Harvey Cushing called the "common devotion" that should motivate the medical profession.[29]

3. *Self-Effacement*

Self-effacement is such an important topic that we devote a chapter to it in our earlier book containing philosophical analysis of the virtues in medicine.[30] Here we may briefly sketch its importance from a religious point of a view.

From the Christian perspective, self-effacement is an obligation of charity toward others, motivated by love and without the motive of self-interest. Few physicians are expected to practice heroic levels of self-sacrifice. But a Christian physician has a moral obligation to be compassionate, considerate, and courteous even to his difficult patients, to be available to them even at some considerable inconvenience to self and to be solicitous for their needs. The Christian perspective precludes some of the excessive expressions of self-pity we see today on the part of physicians—the complaints about income, work hours, delayed gratification, or the justification for recreation at the expense of commitment to patient needs. It precludes also the attitude of some physicians who feel that having worked so hard and paid so much for a medical education, they are entitled to get it back financially or in prestige, privileges, and prerogatives.

Self-effacement, it must be said, however binding it may be in naturalistic and Christocentric medical ethics, does not require neglect of one's personal or familial well-being. Physicians are entitled to develop and grow as persons, to enjoy recreation, to serve their families and provide for their own material needs. Moderate and extreme interpretations of the obligation to self-effacement can be as morally unsound as its neglect. Indeed, immoderate self-sacrifice is too often an excuse for an inability to balance conflicting obligations or even for deliberately neglecting some of them.

The issue is really one of balance, for which no instant formula is at hand, since knowing when legitimate self-interest should dominate, and when self-effacement, is the product of constant reflection and emotional maturity. Suffice it to say that prudence, the virtue St. Thomas thought so central to the Christian life, is the virtue to be cultivated here.[31]

CONCLUSION

The concept of Christian personalism meshes closely with the perspective on the theological virtues we have explored in this book. After all, any virtue-based theory of ethics concentrates on the kind of person the moral agent ought to be. The natural virtues, we argued in our earlier book, define the character traits that enable the physician to aim at excellence in pursuit of the goals of medicine. As the person develops in the profession, the natural virtues fulfill the person through his or her duties as a physician.

Similarly, the Christian virtues seek to define the kind of person the physician ought to be to fulfill his or her calling both as a physician and as a Christian. In this case of the theological virtues, the end sought is itself supernatural because it is instilled by grace in the person, living in accord with the good news of salvation and love. By these virtues the physician attains salvation, not just medical or personal fulfillment. Yet the actions are the same as those of the naturally virtuous physician. The difference lies in expectations. Living a life of charity requires that we love every neighbor, even those who do ill to us or harm us. This is not required of the natural virtues, although kindness toward one's enemies might be laudable and honorable in any event. The Christian physician is be expected to charitably pursue healing.

Another way to put this is that through sin came a separation or rift between the spiritual and the physical in human life. Sin darkened our perception of the integral whole that human beings and, indeed, communal and environmental life ought to be. The natural virtues cannot guarantee the vision required to reintegrate the person and the world itself. Sometimes this is discovered, but only after a long time and very arduously, as St. Thomas Aquinas claimed when discussing the need for faith.[32] The vision the Christian virtues provide and the impetus to act on that vision are truly a grace, a gift. For it provides clarity about the goals and mission of the human person and human society, which are the subject of contentious secular debate.

The emerging contemporary idea of Christian personalism, with its enrichment of the ancient notion of personhood, unites all the elements necessary for both physician and patient to attain the earthly goals of healing and the heavenly goal of the beatific vision.

NOTES

1. Albert Camus, "The Unbeliever and Christians," in *Resistance, Rebellion, and Death* (New York: Alfred A. Knopf, 1961), p. 70.

2. Alasdair MacIntyre, *After Virtue* (Notre Dame: Notre Dame University Press, 1984).

3. Plato, *The Symposium*, trans. Michael Joyce, in *Plato: The Collected Dialogues*, ed. Edith Hamilton and Huntington Cairns (Princeton: Princeton University Press, 1985), 207d, p. 559.

4. The Monophysites—the one "physis" or one nature party—were followers of Eutyches, a monk from Constantinople, who taught that Christ had but one complete nature. Cf. Philip Hughes, *The Church in Crisis: A History of the General Councils 325–1870* (Garden City, N.Y.: Hanover House, 1964), pp. 68ff.

5. Boethius, *De Duabus Naturis et Una Persona Christi* [Patrologia Latina, vol. 64] (Migne, 1860), p. 1343(D).

6. Étienne Gilson, *The Spirit of Medieval Philosophy* (New York: Scribners, 1940), p. 204.

7. Mieczylaw A. Krapiec, *I-Man: An Outline of Philosophical Anthropology,* trans. Marie Lescoe et al. (New Britain, Conn.: Mariel, 1983), pp. 313–333.

8. Karol Wojtyla, *The Acting Person,* trans. Andrezej Potoski (Dordrecht, Netherlands: D. Reidel, 1979), pp. 149–181 and 295–299; Pope John Paul II, *Crossing the Threshold of Hope* (New York: Alfred Knopf, 1994).

9. Pope John Paul II, *Crossing the Threshold,* pp. 200–201.

10. Pope John Paul II, *Crossing the Threshold,* p. 80.

11. Pope John Paul II, *Crossing the Threshold,* p. 201.

12. Pope John Paul II, *Crossing the Threshold,* p. 201.

13. Pope John Paul II, *Encyclical Letter: Veritatis Splendor* (Vatican City: Libreria Editrice Vaticana, 1993), sec. 102, p. 152.

14. Pope John Paul II, *Veritatis Splendor,* sec. 96, p. 145.

15. Ronald Modras, "The Moral Philosophy of Pope John Paul II," *Theological Studies* 41 (December 1980): 683–697; See also pertinent articles in *Proceedings of the American Catholic Philosophical Association* 60 (1986); and Franz Bockle, "Nature as the Basis for Morality," in *Personalist Morals,* ed. Joseph A. Selling (Leuven, Belgium: Leuven University Press, 1988), pp. 51–58.

16. Edmund D. Pellegrino, "Character, Virtue, and Self-Interest in the Ethics of the Professions," *Journal of Contemporary Health Law and Policy* 5 (spring 1989): 53–73.

17. Joseph Spoerl, "Impartiality and the Great Commandment: A Reply to Joseph Cottingham (and Others)," *American Catholic Philosophical Quarterly* 68, no. 2 (1994): 205; St. Thomas Aquinas, *Summa Theologiae* [Vol. 33], trans. and ed. T. R. Heath (New York: Blackfriars, 1972), II-II, q.44, a.7, pp. 154–156.

18. National Institutes of Health, *Report of the Human Embryo Research Panel,* September 27, 1994; Congregation for the Doctrine of the Faith, *Instruction on Respect for Human Life in Its Origin and on the Dignity of Procreation: Replies to Certain Questions of the Day (Donum Vitae)* (Washington: U.S. Catholic Conference, 1987).

19. James T. Burtchaell, "Statement," in *Report of the Human Fetal Tissue Transplantation Research Panel to the Director, National Institutes of Health* [Vol. 1], ed. Consultants to the Advisory Committee to the Director, National Institutes of Health, December 14, 1988, pp. 23–24; Peter J. Cataldo and Albert S. Moraczewski, eds., *The Fetal Tissue Issue: Medical and Ethical Aspects* (Braintree, Mass.: Pope John XXIII Center, 1994).

20. National Institutes of Health, *Report of the Human Embryo Research Panel.*

21. Joseph Daniel Cassidy, O.P., and Edmund D. Pellegrino, "A Catholic

Perspective on Human Gene Therapy," *International Journal of Bioethics* 4, no. 1 (1993): 11–17.

22. Ray G. Frey, "Moral Standing, the Value of Lives and Speciesism," *Between the Species* 4, no. 3 (1988): 191–201. See also Ray G. Frey, *Rights, Killing, and Suffering* (Oxford: Basil Blackwell, 1983).

23. John Lachs, "Active Euthanasia: Theoretical Aspects," *Journal of Clinical Ethics* 1, no. 2 (1990): 113–115.

24. The Oregon Death with Dignity Act, 1994.

25. Ivan Illich, *Medical Nemesis* (New York: Bantam Books, 1977).

26. Edmund D. Pellegrino and David C. Thomasma, *For the Patient's Good: Toward the Restoration of Beneficence in Health Care* (New York: Oxford University Press, 1988), pp. 83–91.

27. William F. May, *The Physician's Covenant* (Philadelphia: Westminster Press, 1983); Pedro L. Entralgo, *La relacion medico-enfermo: Historia y teoria* (Madrid: Revista de Occidente, 1964), pp. 235–258; and Edmund D. Pellegrino, "Toward a Reconstruction of Medical Morality: The Primacy of the Act of Profession and the Fact of Illness," *Journal of Medicine and Philosophy* 4, no. 1 (1979): 32–56.

28. See James Childress' discussion of strong and weak paternalism in his *Who Should Decide? Paternalism in Health Care* (New York: Oxford University Press, 1982), pp. 102–112.

29. Harvey Cushing, "The Common Devotion," in *Consecratio Medici and Other Papers* (Boston: Little, Brown, 1929), pp. 3–13.

30. Edmund D. Pellegrino and David C. Thomasma, *The Virtues in Medical Practice* (New York: Oxford University Press, 1993).

31. Josef Pieper, *The Four Cardinal Virtues* (Notre Dame: University of Notre Dame Press, 1966); St. Thomas Aquinas, *Summa Theologiae* [Vol. 36], trans. and ed. Thomas Gilby (New York: Blackfriars, 1974), II-II, q. 47, a. 4–5, pp. 14–21.

32. Thomas Gilby, general preface to St. Thomas Aquinas, *Summa Theologiae* [Vol. 1], ed. Thomas Gilby (New York: Blackfriars, 1964), p. xi.

Name Index

Subject Index

CPSIA information can be obtained at www.ICGtesting.com
Printed in the USA
BVOW04*1442061214

377805BV00001B/3/P